NURSING DATASOURCE 1995

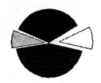

Volume I **Trends in Contemporary Nursing Education**

Pub. No. 19-6649

Division of Research

NATIONAL LEAGUE FOR NURSING

RT79
.N86x
1995
vol. 1

PREFACE

Welcome to the comprehensive **Nursing DataSource 1995, Volume I**—a summation of findings from NLN's Annual Survey of Nursing Education Programs. Volume I, *Trends in Contemporary Nursing Education*, focuses on RN education programs. I am sure you will find the variety and depth of data and analysis presented in **Nursing DataSource 1995** a valuable resource for your own research needs. This volume is especially important for all of us to review and analyze carefully as we transform nursing education to match the changing face of health care.

The following Executive Summary highlights the trends that are emerging in this already changing system of care, explains the reasons for these trends, and anticipates what we can expect in the future. The pages of tables, graphs, and charts clearly expand upon this general analysis for further understanding and extrapolation of data.

NLN Research has continued to grow and expand to match a profession whose needs are many and whose future is invaluable to healthy communities. I'm sure you'll agree as you discover the wealth of information provided in **Nursing DataSource 1995, Volume I**.

Patricia Moccia, PhD, RN, FAAN
Chief Executive Officer
National League for Nursing
NLN RESEARCH

ABOUT THE DIVISION

Nursing DataSource 1995 is a summary of data collected from the National League for Nursing's Annual Survey of Nursing Education Programs. Since 1953, NLN Research has been maintaining and updating a comprehensive data bank on all state-approved nursing education programs. The Nursing DataSource series contains a vast array of trend analysis, in terms of nursing education programs, student admissions, enrollments, graduations and ethnic background. Nursing DataSource Volume I focuses on RN programs; Volume II focuses on graduate nursing programs; and Volume III focuses on PN/VN programs. The survey results are widely used by government officials, nurse educators, policy makers, consultants, and others interested in health care and the future supply and demand for nurses.

NLN's Annual Survey is conducted with a sophisticated research design and rigorous data collection methodology. Each year, with the cooperation of each state board of nursing, NLN Research surveys the more than 3,000 nursing education programs in operation within the United States. It includes all PN/VN, diploma, associate degree, baccalaureate, master's and doctoral programs. A 100 percent response rate has been maintained in the areas of admissions, enrollments and graduations. Response rates of approximately 85 percent have been achieved for data on men and minorities, tuition, and other variables.

NLN Research is also exploring new opportunities to create a dialogue with members of the research community. To accomplish this, NLN Research has initiated the following programs:

Seminars—NLN has brought together intimate groups of major thinkers to discuss contemporary issues and set direction for policy, planning, and implementation. The First Annual Research Institute held in August, 1995 focused on community-based nursing and public health. In 1996, NLN Research will expand the series to provide an introductory level for new nurse researchers, and an advanced level for senior researchers and policy analysts.

Training—NLN welcomes pre- and post-doctoral students from the fields of nursing, sociology, psychology, and epidemiology. In 1995, NLN welcomed two faculty members from Thailand who received training in research methodology. In 1996, faculty from South Africa and England will also visit.

Internships—NLN offers internships to provide meaningful research experiences that will foster the development of the next generation of health researchers. The interns can have access to NLN Research's database, or use data which they have collected, to provide them with hand-on experience in statistical analysis.

Other publications by NLN Research include *Profiles of the Newly Licensed Nurse, 3rd edition*, which will summarize the results from the 1994 Newly Licensed Nurse Survey, and the *1995 Nurse Educators*, which will summarize the results from the 1994 Nurse Faculty Census Survey. We also have a new publication, *Annual Guide to Graduate Nursing Education 1995*, which lists all master's and doctoral nursing education programs in the country. In addition, NLN Research publishes *PRISM*, a quarterly newsletter which provides an in-depth analysis of a single topic related to health care, education and other contemporary concerns. Recent issues focused on nursing education in changing times, and community-based care.

For further information about other publications and products from NLN Research, as well as current activities, call 212-989-9393, ext. 160, or use our internet address: nlninform@nln.org.

Delroy Louden PhD
Vice President
NLN Research

Table of Contents

Preface iii
About the Division of Research iv

SECTION I
   EXECUTIVE SUMMARY 1

SECTION 2
   GRAPHS 9
   Figure 1
      OVERALL ENROLLMENTS DECLINED
      FOR THE FIRST TIME IN SIX YEARS 11
   Figure 2
      ENROLLMENTS INCREASED IN BASIC BACCALAUREATE PROGRAMS
      BUT DECREASED IN ASSOCIATE DEGREE
      AND DIPLOMA PROGRAMS 11
   Figure 3
      RN ENROLLMENTS INTO BASIC BACCALAUREATE
      PROGRAMS INCREASE BY 10.7 PERCENT 12
   Figure 4
      MAJORITY OF RN STUDENTS ATTENDED SCHOOL PART-TIME 12
   Figure 5
      OVERALL FALL ADMISSIONS
      DECLINED FOR THE FIRST TIME IN SIX YEARS 13
   Figure 6
      FALL ADMISSIONS INCREASE ONLY
      AT BASIC BACCALAUREATE PROGRAMS 13
   Figure 7
      NUMBER OF DIPLOMA PROGRAMS CONTINUED TO DECLINE 14
   Figure 8
      DROP IN THE NUMBER OF APPLICATIONS
      TO ASSOCIATE DEGREE AND DIPLOMA PROGRAMS 14

Figure 9
   ANNUAL ADMISSIONS INCREASED IN
   BASIC BACCALAUREATE AND ASSOCIATE DEGREE PROGRAMS 15
Figure 10
   GRADUATIONS INCREASED FROM ALL BASIC RN PROGRAMS 15
Figure 11
   MODEST INCREASE IN PERCENTAGE OF
   MINORITY STUDENTS ENROLLED IN NURSING PROGRAMS 16
Figure 12
   STEADY INCREASE IN THE PERCENTAGE OF
   MEN GRADUATING FROM NURSING PROGRAMS 16
Figure 13
   MAJORITY OF BASIC BACCLAUREATE PROGRAMS OFFERED
   BOTH SPECIFIC AND INTEGRATED COURSES
   ON COMMUNITY-BASED CARE 17
Figure 14
   THE VAST MAJORITY OF NURSING PROGRAMS USE
   COMMUNITY-BASED CARE SETTINGS AS CLINICAL SITES 17

SECTION 3

Numeric Tables 19
Table 1
   BASIC RN PROGRAMS AND PERCENTAGE CHANGE FROM
   PREVIOUS YEAR, BY TYPE OF PROGRAM: 1974 TO 1994 21
Table 2
   PUBLIC AND PRIVATE BASIC RN PROGRAMS,
   BY TYPE OF PROGRAM: 1985 TO 1994 21
Table 3
   ALL BASIC RN PROGRAMS,
   BY NLN REGION AND STATE: 1985 TO 1994 22
Table 4
   BASIC BACCALAUREATE NURSING PROGRAMS,
   BY NLN REGION AND STATE: 1985 TO 1994 23
Table 5
   ASSOCIATE DEGREE NURSING PROGRAMS,
   BY NLN REGION AND STATE: 1985 TO 1994 24
Table 6
   DIPLOMA NURSING PROGRAMS,
   BY NLN REGION AND STATE: 1985 TO 1994 25
Table 7
   BACCALAUREATE NURSING PROGRAMS THAT ENROLL BASIC
   AND/OR RN STUDENTS, BY NLN ACCREDITATION STATUS:
   JANUARY, 1995 26

Table 8
BASIC RN PROGRAMS, BY TYPE OF PROGRAM AND NLN
ACCREDITATION STATUS: JANUARY, 1995 27
Table 9
MEAN ANNUAL TUITIONS OF FULL-TIME STUDENTS IN PUBLIC OR
PRIVATE BASIC RN PROGRAMS: 1994 TO 1995 28
Table 10
FALL ADMISSIONS TO PUBLIC AND PRIVATE BASIC RN PROGRAMS,
BY TYPE OF PROGRAM: 1985 TO 1994 28
Table 11
ANNUAL ADMISSIONS TO BASIC RN PROGRAMS AND PERCENTAGE
CHANGE FROM PREVIOUS YEAR, BY TYPE OF PROGRAM:
1974-75 TO 1993-94 29
Table 12
ANNUAL ADMISSIONS TO PUBLIC AND PRIVATE BASIC RN
PROGRAMS, BY TYPE OF PROGRAM: 1984-85 TO 1993-94 29
Table 13
ANNUAL ADMISSIONS TO ALL BASIC RN PROGRAMS,
BY NLN REGION AND STATE: 1984-85 TO 1993-94 30
Table 14
ANNUAL ADMISSIONS TO BASIC BACCALAUREATE NURSING
PROGRAMS, BY NLN REGION AND STATE: 1984-85 TO 1993-94 31
Table 15
ANNUAL ADMISSIONS TO ASSOCIATE DEGREE NURSING
PROGRAMS, BY NLN REGION AND STATE: 1984-85 TO 1993-94 32
Table 16
ANNUAL ADMISSIONS TO DIPLOMA NURSING PROGRAMS,
BY NLN REGION AND STATE: 1984-85 TO 1993-94 33
Table 17
ENROLLMENTS IN BASIC RN PROGRAMS AND PERCENTAGE CHANGE
FROM PREVIOUS YEAR, BY TYPE OF PROGRAM: 1975 TO 1994 34
Table 18
ENROLLMENTS IN PUBLIC AND PRIVATE BASIC RN PROGRAMS,
BY TYPE OF PROGRAM: 1985 TO 1994 34
Table 19
TOTAL ENROLLMENTS IN ALL BASIC RN PROGRAMS,
BY NLN REGION AND STATE: 1985 TO 1994 35
Table 20
TOTAL ENROLLMENTS IN BASIC BACCALAUREATE NURSING
PROGRAMS, BY NLN REGION AND STATE: 1985 TO 1994 36
Table 21
TOTAL ENROLLMENTS IN ASSOCIATE DEGREE NURSING PROGRAMS,
BY NLN REGION AND STATE: 1985 TO 1994 37

Table 22
TOTAL ENROLLMENTS IN DIPLOMA NURSING PROGRAMS,
BY NLN REGION AND STATE: 1985 TO 1994 38
Table 23
BASIC AND RN STUDENT ENROLLMENTS IN BACCALAUREATE
NURSING PROGRAMS: 1985 TO 1994 39
Table 24
FULL-TIME AND PART-TIME ENROLLMENTS OF BASIC AND RN
STUDENTS IN BACCALAUREATE NURSING PROGRAMS:
1990 TO 1994 39
Table 25
TOTAL ENROLLMENTS IN BACCALAUREATE NURSING PROGRAMS,
BY NLN REGION AND STATE: 1990 TO 1994 40
Table 26
GRADUATIONS FROM BASIC RN PROGRAMS AND PERCENTAGE
CHANGE FROM PREVIOUS YEAR, BY TYPE OF PROGRAM:
1974-75 TO 1993-94 41
Table 27
GRADUATIONS FROM PUBLIC AND PRIVATE BASIC RN PROGRAMS,
BY TYPE OF PROGRAM: 1984-85 TO 1993-94 .41
Table 28
GRADUATIONS FROM ALL BASIC RN PROGRAMS,
BY NLN REGION AND STATE: 1984-85 TO 1993-94 42
Table 29
GRADUATIONS FROM BASIC BACCALAUREATE NURSING PROGRAMS,
BY NLN REGION AND STATE: 1984-85 TO 1993-94 43
Table 30
GRADUATIONS FROM ASSOCIATE DEGREE NURSING PROGRAMS,
BY NLN REGION AND STATE: 1984-85 TO 1993-94 44
Table 31
GRADUATIONS FROM DIPLOMA NURSING PROGRAMS,
BY NLN REGION AND STATE: 1984-85 TO 1993-94 45
Table 32
BASIC AND RN STUDENT GRADUATIONS FROM BACCALAUREATE
NURSING PROGRAMS: 1984-85 TO 1993-94 46
Table 33
GRADUATIONS OF REGISTERED NURSES FROM BACCALAUREATE
NURSING PROGRAMS, BY PREVIOUS BASIC NURSING EDUCATION AND
REGION: 1989-90 TO 1993-94 46
Table 34
TOTAL GRADUATIONS FROM BACCALAUREATE NURSING PROGRAMS,
BY NLN REGION AND STATE: 1990 TO 1994 47
Table 35
APPLICATIONS PER FALL ADMISSION FOR BASIC RN PROGRAMS,
BY TYPE OF PROGRAM AND NLN REGION: 1994 48

Table 36

    PERCENTAGE OF APPLICATIONS FOR ADMISSION ACCEPTED AND NOT
    ACCEPTED AND PERCENTAGE ON WAITING LISTS FOR ALL BASIC RN
    PROGRAMS, BY TYPE OF PROGRAM: 1994 48

SECTION 4

Numeric Tables on Male and Minority Students 49

Table 1

    ESTIMATED NUMBER OF STUDENT ADMISSIONS TO ALL BASIC RN
    PROGRAMS, BY RACE/ETHNICITY, NLN REGION AND STATE:
    1993-1994 51

Table 2

    ESTIMATED NUMBER OF STUDENT ADMISSIONS TO BASIC
    BACCALAUREATE NURSING PROGRAMS, BY RACE/ETHNICITY, NLN
    REGION AND STATE: 1993-1994 52

Table 3

    ESTIMATED NUMBER OF STUDENT ADMISSIONS TO ASSOCIATE
    DEGREE NURSING PROGRAMS, BY RACE/ETHNICITY,
    NLN REGION AND STATE: 1993-1994 53

Table 4

    ESTIMATED NUMBER OF STUDENT ADMISSIONS TO DIPLOMA
    NURSING PROGRAMS, BY RACE/ETHNICITY, NLN REGION AND STATE:
    1993-1994 54

Table 5

    TRENDS IN THE ESTIMATED NUMBER OF ANNUAL ADMISSIONS
    OF MINORITY STUDENTS TO BASIC RN PROGRAMS,
    1988-89 TO 1993-94 55

Table 6

    ESTIMATED NUMBER OF STUDENT ENROLLMENTS
    IN ALL BASIC RN PROGRAMS, BY RACE/ETHNICITY, NLN REGION AND
    STATE: 1994 56

Table 7

    ESTIMATED NUMBER OF STUDENT ENROLLMENTS IN BASIC
    BACCALAUREATE NURSING PROGRAMS, BY RACE/ETHNICITY,
    NLN REGION AND STATE: 1994 57

Table 8

    ESTIMATED NUMBER OF STUDENT ENROLLMENTS IN ASSOCIATE
    DEGREE NURSING PROGRAMS, BY RACE/ETHNICITY,
    NLN REGION AND STATE: 1994 58

Table 9

    ESTIMATED NUMBER OF STUDENT ENROLLMENTS IN DIPLOMA
    NURSING PROGRAMS, BY RACE/ETHNICITY,
    NLN REGION AND STATE: 1994 59

Table 10
TRENDS IN THE ESTIMATED NUMBER OF ENROLLMENTS
OF MINORITY STUDENTS IN BASIC RN PROGRAMS, 1989 TO 1994 . . . 60
Table 11
ESTIMATED NUMBER OF STUDENT GRADUATIONS FROM ALL BASIC
RN PROGRAMS, BY RACE/ETHNICITY, NLN REGION AND STATE: 1993-
1994 61
Table 12
ESTIMATED NUMBER OF STUDENT GRADUATIONS FROM BASIC
BACCALAUREATE NURSING PROGRAMS, BY RACE/ETHNICITY, NLN
REGION AND STATE: 1993-1994 62
Table 13
ESTIMATED NUMBER OF STUDENT GRADUATIONS FROM ASSOCIATE
DEGREE NURSING PROGRAMS, BY RACE/ETHNICITY, NLN REGION AND
STATE: 1993-1994 63
Table 14
ESTIMATED NUMBER OF STUDENT GRADUATIONS FROM DIPLOMA
NURSING PROGRAMS, BY RACE/ETHNICITY,
NLN REGION AND STATE: 1993-1994 64
Table 15
TRENDS IN THE ESTIMATED NUMBER OF GRADUATIONS OF MINORITY
STUDENTS FROM BASIC RN PROGRAMS, 1988-89 TO 1993-94 65
Table 16
ADMISSIONS OF MEN TO ALL BASIC RN PROGRAMS,
BY NLN REGION: 1993-1994 66
Table 17
TRENDS IN ADMISSIONS OF MEN TO ALL BASIC RN PROGRAMS:
1984-1994 66
Table 18
ENROLLMENTS OF MEN IN ALL BASIC RN PROGRAMS,
BY NLN REGION: 1994 67
Table 19
TRENDS IN ENROLLMENTS OF MEN
IN ALL BASIC RN PROGRAMS: 1984-1994 67
Table 20
GRADUATIONS OF MEN FROM ALL BASIC RN PROGRAMS,
BY NLN REGION: 1993-1994 68
Table 21
TRENDS IN GRADUATIONS OF MEN FROM ALL BASIC RN PROGRAMS:
1984-1994 68

Section 1
Executive Summary

EXECUTIVE SUMMARY

OVERALL ENROLLMENTS DECLINED IN 1994
REVERSING A SIX-YEAR TREND

According to the results of the 1994 Annual Survey of RN Programs, overall enrollments declined, reversing a six-year trend (Figure 1). Associate degree enrollments decreased by one percent in 1994, as compared to an increase of 3.5 percent in 1993 (Figure 2). This was the first sign of a reduction in associate degree enrollments since 1986, although these students still comprised over 50 percent of total enrollments. There was also a decline in diploma enrollments for the second year in a row.

An increase in enrollments was limited to basic baccalaureate programs, which experienced a 1.8 percent increase in basic students[1], and a 10.7 percent increase in RNs returning to obtain a baccalaureate degree (Figure 3). The latter finding is of interest because it clearly indicates that current RNs find it advantageous to advance their education at least to the baccalaureate level, which would then allow them to continue on for an advanced degree. In addition, the vast majority of RNs enrolled in basic baccalaureate programs attended part-time, while the great majority of basic students attended full-time (Figure 4). Thus, basic baccalaureate nursing programs must address the needs of this growing segment of their student population.

In 1994, overall fall admissions also declined for the first time in six years, again with the decrease limited to associate degree and diploma programs (Figures 5 & 6). Fall admissions are used as a predictor for future enrollments. In fact, 1993 fall admissions declined for both diploma and associate degree programs, accurately predicting the 1994 decline in enrollments for both program types.

The number of RN programs remained stable for basic baccalaureate programs, and declined for diploma programs (Figure 7). The number of associate degree programs increased by 11. However, there was a drop in the number of applications[2] to associate degree and diploma programs of 11 percent and 18 percent, respectively (Figure 8). In contrast, there was a 4 percent increase for basic baccalaureate programs.

Overall annual admissions[3] increased for the seventh consecutive year, although it was the smallest percentage increase within that time frame (2.4%). The increases occurred in basic baccalaureate and associate degree programs (Figure 9).

Overall graduations increased as well by 7.6 percent. The increase was evident across program types, ranging from 2.6 percent from diploma programs to 18.3 percent from basic baccalaureate programs (Figure 10). These increases resulted from the upward trend in enrollments over the past few years. However, now that the trend in enrollments is reversing, especially for diploma and associate degree programs, it is likely that graduations will begin to fall in these programs as well.

---

[1] Basic students are students who do not hold an RN license.

[2] This is based on programs that reported number of applications and admitted a class in the fall of the survey year.

[3] Admissions are defined as all first-time nursing students who have never been previously enrolled in any RN nursing program.

For the 1994-95 school year, the average annual tuition at public institutions was $1,762 for state residents and $4,399 for non-residents, which was an increase of approximately 5 percent from the 1993-94 school year. The average annual tuition at private institutions was $7,965, which was an increase of approximately 6 percent compared to the 1993-94 school year. Private basic baccalaureate programs had the highest average annual tuition at $9,941, while the lowest tuition was paid by state residents attending associate degree programs, with an average annual tuition of $1,480.

MINORITY ENROLLMENT AND GRADUATION

In general, there were minimal increases between 1993 and 1994 in annual admissions, enrollments and graduations of minority students. Specifically, for annual admissions, the percentage of minority students changed from 15.6 in 1993 to 16.2 in 1994, with a slight increase evident for each minority group.

There was a slight increase in the percentage of minority students enrolled in RN programs, going from 15.7 percent in 1993 to 16.5 percent in 1994. These increases were evident across minority groups, with the exception of American Indians, which remained stable at .7 percent (Figure 11).

There was also a minimal increase in the percentage of minority students who graduated from RN programs between 1993 and 1994, 12.7% and 13.3%, respectively. While the percentage of Hispanic and Asian graduates increased slightly, the percentage of black graduates remained stable, and the percentage of American Indian graduates decreased slightly.

ENROLLMENT OF MEN IN NURSING PROGRAMS

The percentage of men admitted to RN programs stabilized between 1993 and 1994, at least in basic baccalaureate and diploma programs. However, there has been a steady increase in men admitted to associate degree programs, growing from seven percent in 1988 to 14 percent in 1994.

Enrollments of men to RN programs was also stable across program type, with enrollments remaining at 12 percent for basic baccalaureate programs, and approximately 13 percent for associate degree and diploma programs. The only noticeable increase occurred with overall graduations, which grew from 10.5 percent in 1993 to 11.4 percent in 1994 (Figure 12). The greatest increase occurred with diploma programs, where the percentage of male graduates increased from 10.6 percent in 1993 to 12 percent in 1994.

REASONS FOR DECLINING ENROLLMENTS

Declining enrollments may be related to specific characteristics of nursing education, or to more general characteristics of higher education. In terms of nursing education, programs may be voluntarily reducing their enrollments as a reaction to difficulties their graduates face in finding employment. Such difficulties were apparent in the results from the 1994 NLN Newly Licensed Nurse study, a national study of over 61,000 registered nurses who were licensed in July 1993. In the spring of 1994, after nine months of experience in the labor force, these new RNs were surveyed to identify their demographic and educational characteristics, and their employment experiences. In 1990, 83 percent of the respondents reported finding their first job in nursing before graduating the RN program. In 1992 there was little change with 81 percent reporting this. However, in 1994 this dropped to 64 percent. In addition, when asked about their perception of job availability, 63 percent reported many jobs were available in 1990, compared to just 6 percent in 1994.

With respect to the findings from NLN's annual survey, a comparison was made between the admission slots available in 1993 and then in 1994. The mean number of slots available in 1993 as compared to 1994 for basic baccalaureate programs were 74 and 75, respectively; for associate degree programs 75 and 70, respectively; and for diploma programs 72 and 65, respectively.

However, the American Council on Education reported an overall drop in 1994 college enrollments.[1] This was attributed to an overall reduction in college-age students, and a reduction in state appropriations which has resulted in increased tuition, reduced course offerings, and a limit in the number of students served. It is unlikely that decreased enrollments in associate degree programs was the result of a reduction in college-age students, because the mean age of the associate degree respondents to the 1994 Newly Licensed Nurse survey was 34. On the other hand, tuition increases may have had an impact, especially with private rather than public programs.

In an attempt to discern the reason for reduced enrollments, NLN's 1995 Annual Survey includes a question about whether nursing schools have planned to reduce the number of students admitted into the program, and if so, why. Results from this survey are anticipated to be available by June, 1996.

COMMUNITY-BASED CARE AND NURSING EDUCATION

Every year questions are included on NLN's Annual Survey to address current issues in nursing education. The 1994 Annual Survey included a section on community-based care, and the extent the concept was part of the nursing education curriculum. The questions focused on whether the concept was taught in the program, whether it was taught as a specific course or integrated into a general course, and whether community-based care settings were used as clinical sites. In general, community-based care was part of the curriculum at the majority of nursing programs.

According to the results, 75 percent of the RN programs taught the concept of community-based care. In terms of program type, 90 percent of basic baccalaureate, 65 percent of associate degree and 85 percent of diploma programs included the topic in their curricula. The vast majority of associate degree and diploma programs integrated the concept into a general course (Figure 13). In contrast, 21.3 percent of the basic baccalaureate programs offered a specific course, and 53.9 percent offered both a specific course and integrated it into a general course.

More than 80 percent of the RN programs used community-based care settings as clinical sites. In basic baccalaureate and diploma programs, the percentages reached 90 percent, compared to 78 percent in associate degree programs (Figure 14). Overall, nursing homes were cited most often as a clinical site (20.4%), followed by home care agencies (17.7%) and day care centers (14.1%). Sites used least often were HMOs (.1%) and homeless shelters (.7%). These results indicate that nursing education programs are teaching community-based care, both didactically and experientially.

EDUCATION TO EMPLOYMENT:
THE CHANGING PATTERNS OF HOSPITAL SERVICES

Many health care professionals have been slow to recognize the major structural changes in health care, in terms of staff reductions and closing of hospitals, and the proliferation of managed-care settings. These changes are having a profound impact on the medical and nursing profession, with some winners and some losers.

With respect to the medical profession, general practitioners, as compared to specialists, are the winners because tightly managed health care plans use a higher proportion of primary care physicians, with a lesser emphasis placed on specialists.[2] With respect to the nursing profession, while RNs are losing hospital positions because of reduced nursing budgets, advanced practice nurses are increasingly in demand at managed care centers, as part of the mix of primary care specialists.[3,4] For example, HMOs are using them as disease specialists to provide cost-effective services in such areas as obstetrics, AIDS units, home and terminal care.[5] However, there is not a one-to-one relationship between positions lost in hospitals and gained in HMOs.

Thus, some in the profession failed to gather the trend that hospital revenues from in-patient services have been falling as hospitals expanded their ambulatory services, and made shifts or substitutions for the traditional in-patient services in order to meet the aggressive competition for new patients by their competitors. The profession must face up to the changing trends in health care in general, and hospital services in particular, and the consequent declining role of inpatient care. The results from NLN's 1994 Annual Survey indicate that nursing education has recognized this shift, and is including community-based care in the curriculum.

However, quality of patient care should not be allowed to fall in between the cracks as these structural shifts take place. Yet assessing the effects on quality of care is especially difficult due to deficiencies in definitions and measurement tools presently available—a more concentrated effort is needed to refine and validate these measures. In the mean time, it is useful to examine the health care models in other countries to learn from their experiences.

FINANCING AND ORGANIZATION

In the nursing research and health policy community, interest in the experiences of other countries has been largely confined to issues related to how health care systems are financed.

> In general, the assumption is made that it is the difference in methods of financing health systems that explains the large differences in expenditures on health-related care. These analyses hardly address the impact of different organizational characteristics on differences in outcomes of care. This situation is all the more curious, given the diversity of organizational arrangements and the consequent possibilities for exploring their relationship to improvements in the health of populations.[6]

Given the shift in the United States from the process of health service models to outcomes it is instructive to examine international data that analyzes the relationship between certain aspects of the health systems and indicators of outcomes. In a recent paper that examined health indicators and the organization of health care systems, Elola, Daponte and Navarro[7] argued that countries with National Health Systems would be superior in their achievements when compared to countries with National Health Insurance. Countries with National Health Systems, such as Spain, Ireland, Greece, and the United Kingdom, finance the system by general taxation and these systems are publicly managed. On the other hand, National Security Systems (i.e., National Health Insurance Systems) are financed from mandatory payroll withdrawals and are privately managed. France, Switzerland and Germany have National Health Insurance Systems.

Surprisingly, Elola et at.[7] found little difference between the two systems with respect to life expectancy or potential years of life lost. On the other hand, when they controlled for the effects of gross national product and health care expenditure, which were higher in countries with National Health Insurance Systems, *infant mortality* alone stood out as being lower in countries with National Health Systems. In addition, with each unit increase in health expenditures, there was a greater reduction in infant mortality in countries with National Health Systems, as compared to countries with National Health Insurance Systems.

Obviously, the central question posed by these findings is why infant mortality, as an indicator, differentiates the two systems as compared to other indicators such as life expectancy or years of life lost? Further, how does the financing of services impact the effectiveness of such services? Put simply, why is it that mortality seems more sensitive at such an early age in National Health Systems models as compared to National Health Insurance Systems?

Some answers can be found in the study by Starfield[8] which contrasts the findings of Elola et al.[7] on financing mechanisms with comparative data from eleven countries ranked on fourteen indicators of health: infant mortality and its two components (neonatal and post-neonatal mortality): life expectancy at age one, age 10, age 65 and age 80 each for males and females separately; years of potential life lost; age adjusted death rate; and low birth weight ratio. The criteria outlined by Elola et al.[7] resulted in six countries with National Insurance Systems (Belgium, Canada, Australia, the United States, the Netherlands, and Germany), and five countries with National Health Systems (Denmark, Spain, Finland, Sweden and the United Kingdom). On average, countries with National Health Systems ranked higher, i.e., had lower infant mortality rates, than countries with National Health Insurance Systems, 4.95 and 6.88, respectively. However, countries did not differ in the ranking of indicators at other ages (6.02 for countries with National Health Insurance Systems versus 6.11 for countries with National Health Systems), thus clearly supporting the findings of Elola et al.[7] that the benefit from National Health Systems was confined to infant mortality.

However, Starfield[6] subsequently re-examined these eleven countries based on the strength of their primary care structures, rather than how the structure was financed. The countries were re-categorized according to the following characteristics: coordination of care; reimbursement; first contact; comprehensiveness; community and orientation. Significant differences appeared for all indicators, in addition to other outcome indicators, e.g., satisfaction with care, and medication use. Specifically, countries characterized as providing a strong infrastructure of primary care services were rated significantly higher on a variety of health indicators across the age span. Additionally, there was a relationship between primary care and mode of financing services (e.g., countries with a strong primary care focus were more likely to be National Health Systems than National Health Insurance Systems). The exception was the Netherlands, which has an excellent National Health Insurance financing system, but at the same time a very good primary care system. "Despite the apparent importance of primary care as a major contribution to improved health status, it is useful to remember that primary care may be only a marker for social systems that focus on achieving equity in the distribution of health and social services in general."[6]

Finally, in light of the move to managed care we need to ask the following question, "To what extent does the person-focused relationship, as evidence in the British general practitioners role, enhance the effectiveness and continuity of care?" The evidence from Hjortdahl[9] showed that a period of two years was required for a stable and satisfactory relationship to be established. Clearly managed care that requires patients to shift their source of care when insurance management changes are unlikely to meet the goals of primary care as presently experienced. One way around this conundrum is to achieve better integration of facilities and services.

Delroy Louden, PhD
Vice President, NLN Research

Donna Post, PhD
Research Coordinator, NLN Research

REFERENCES

1. American Council on Education. (1995). States report declines in college enrollments. *Higher Education & National Affairs, 44* (1), pp. 1, 5.

2. Reinhardt, U.E. (1994). Planning the nation's health workforce: Let the market in. *Inquiry, 31*(3), 250-263.

3. Magnusson, P. (1995, October 23). When medicare is reshuffled, who will hold the aces? *Business Week*, p. 33.

4. Survey finds loss of RNs jeopardizes patient safely. (1995). *The American Nurse, 27*(1), pp. 1, 6.

5. Moore, G.T. (1994). Will the power of the marketplace produce the workforce we need? *Inquiry, 31*(3), 276-282.

6. Starfield, B. (1995). Health systems effects on health status-Financing versus organization of services. *American Journal of Public Health, 85* (10), 1350-1351.

7. Elola, J., Daponte, A., & Navarro, V. (1995). Health indicators and the organization of health care systems in Western Europe. *American Journal of Public Health, 85,* 1397-1401.

8. Starfield, B. (1992). *Primary care: Concept, evaluation and policy.* New York: Oxford University Press.

9. Hjortdahl, P. (1992). Continuity of care: General practitioners knowledge about and sense of responsibility towards their patients. *Family Practitioner, 9,* 3-8.

Section 2
Graphs

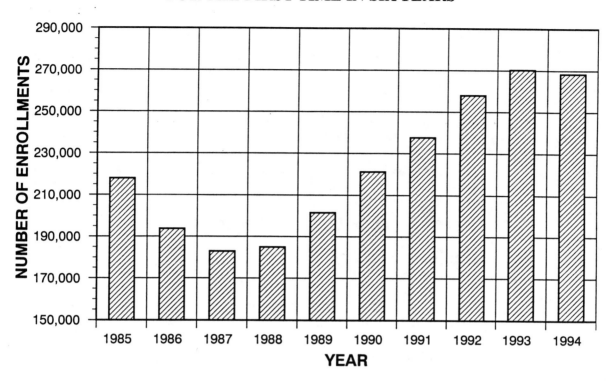

Figure 1
OVERALL ENROLLMENTS DECLINED
FOR THE FIRST TIME IN SIX YEARS

Figure 2
ENROLLMENTS INCREASED IN BASIC BACCALAUREATE PROGRAMS
BUT DECREASED IN ASSOCIATE DEGREE AND DIPLOMA PROGRAMS

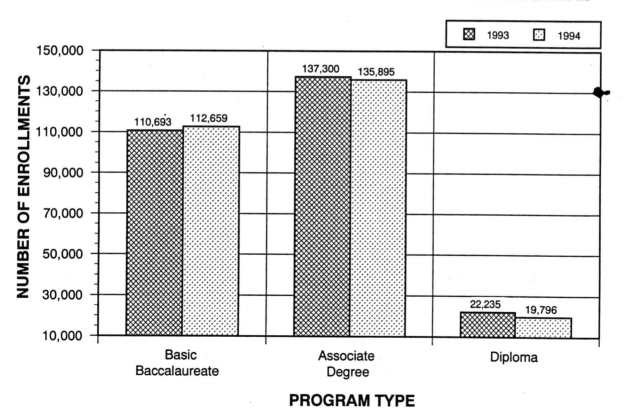

Figure 3
RN ENROLLMENTS INTO BASIC BACCALAUREATE
PROGRAMS INCREASE BY 10.7 PERCENT

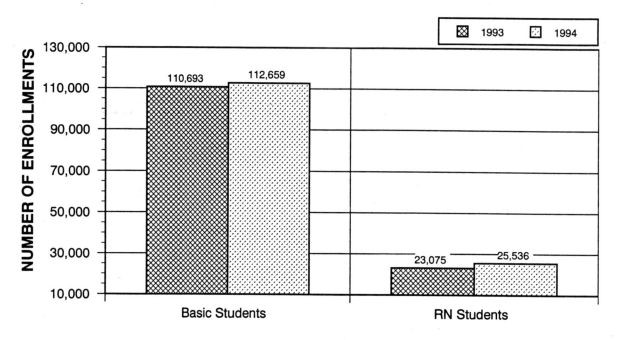

TYPE OF BASIC BACCALAUREATE STUDENT

Figure 4
MAJORITY OF RN STUDENTS ATTENDED SCHOOL PART-TIME

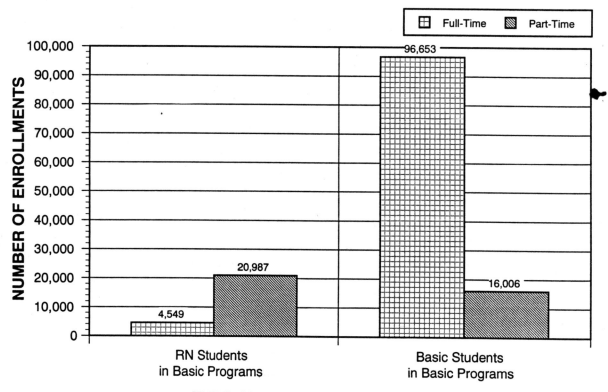

TYPE OF BACCALAUREATE STUDENTS

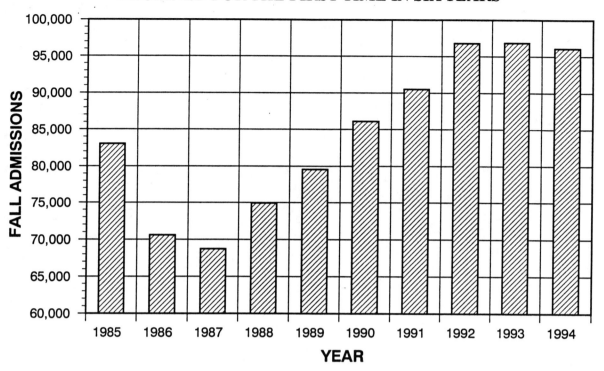

Figure 5
OVERALL FALL ADMISSIONS
DECLINED FOR THE FIRST TIME IN SIX YEARS

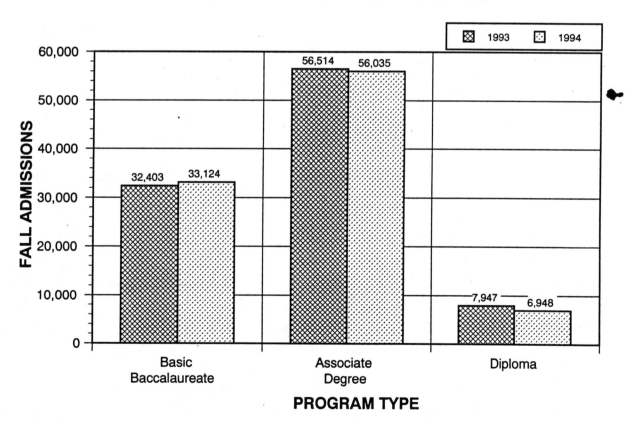

Figure 6
FALL ADMISSIONS INCREASE ONLY
AT BASIC BACCALAUREATE PROGRAMS

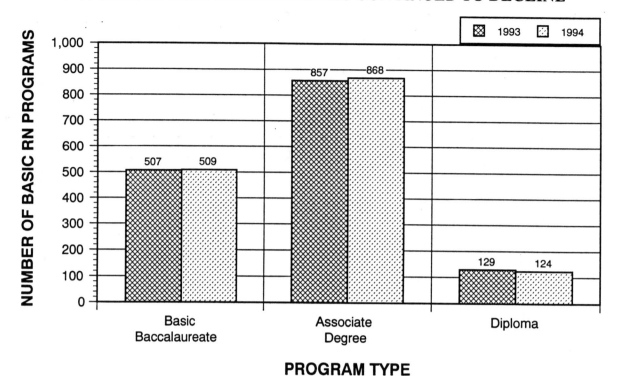

Figure 7
NUMBER OF DIPLOMA PROGRAMS CONTINUED TO DECLINE

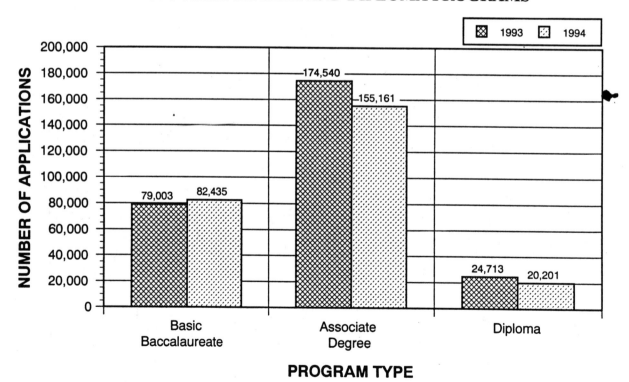

Figure 8
DROP IN THE NUMBER OF APPLICATIONS
TO ASSOCIATE DEGREE AND DIPLOMA PROGRAMS

* Includes programs that reported number of applications, and admitted a class in the fall of the survey year.

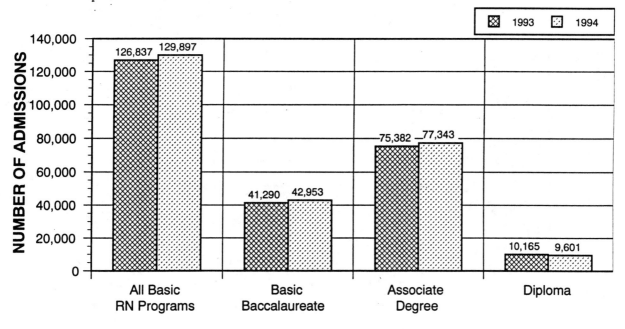

Figure 9
ANNUAL ADMISSIONS INCREASED IN
BASIC BACCALAUREATE AND ASSOCIATE DEGREE PROGRAMS

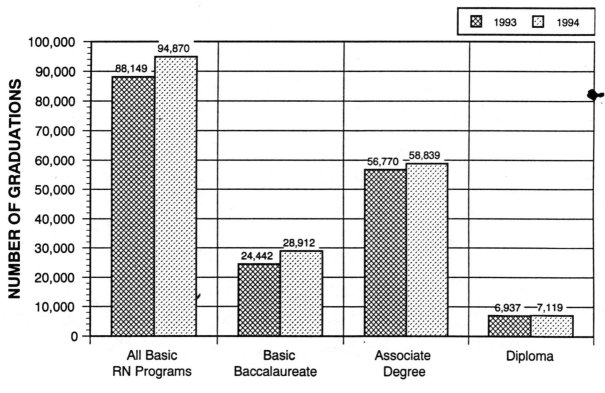

Figure 10
GRADUATIONS INCREASED FROM ALL BASIC RN PROGRAMS

Figure 11
MODEST INCREASE IN PERCENTAGE OF
MINORITY STUDENTS ENROLLED IN NURSING PROGRAMS

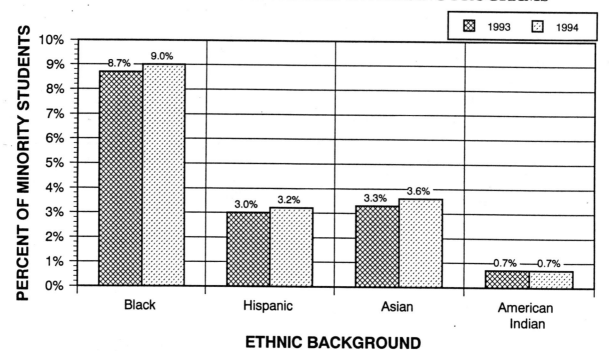

Figure 12
STEADY INCREASE IN THE PERCENTAGE OF
MEN GRADUATING FROM NURSING PROGRAMS

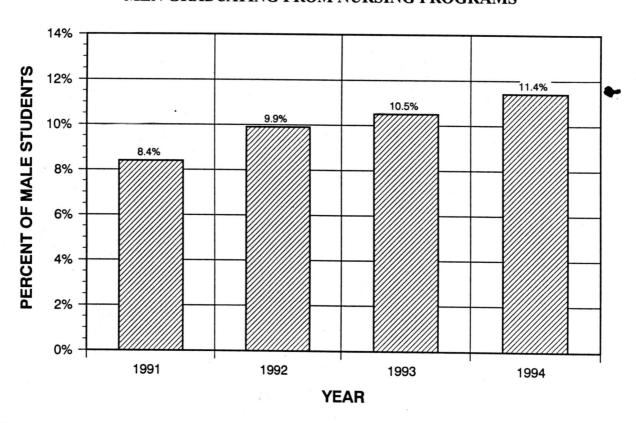

16

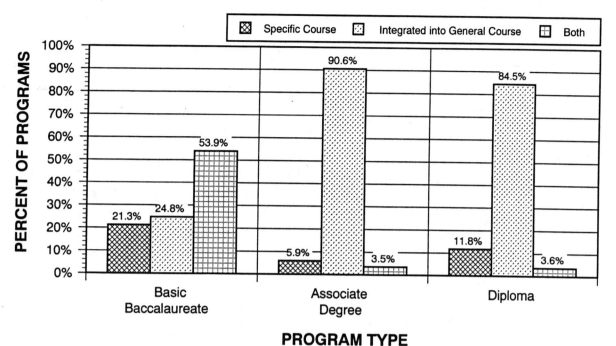

Figure 13
MAJORITY OF BASIC BACCLAUREATE PROGRAMS OFFERED BOTH SPECIFIC AND INTEGRATED COURSES ON COMMUNITY-BASED CARE

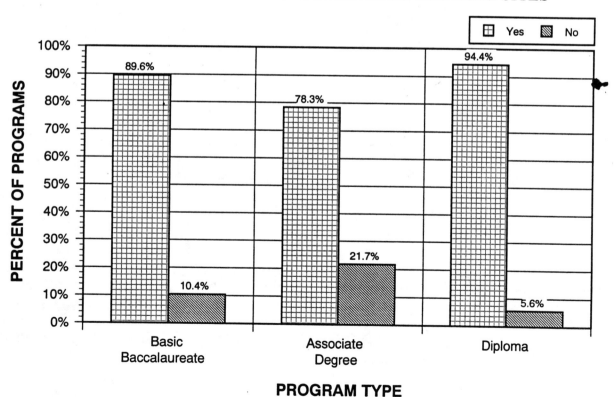

Figure 14
THE VAST MAJORITY OF NURSING PROGRAMS USE COMMUNITY-BASED CARE SETTINGS AS CLINICAL SITES

17

Section 3
Numeric Tables

Table 1
**BASIC RN PROGRAMS AND PERCENTAGE CHANGE FROM PREVIOUS YEAR,
BY TYPE OF PROGRAM: 1974 TO 1994[1]**

YEAR	NUMBER OF SCHOOLS	ALL BASIC RN PROGRAMS		BACCALAUREATE PROGRAMS		ASSOCIATE DEGREE PROGRAMS		DIPLOMA PROGRAMS	
		Number of Programs	Percent Change	Number of Programs	Percent Change	Number of Programs	Percent Change	Number of Programs	Percent Change
1974	1,347	1,358	-0.1	310	+2.6	588	+4.1	460	-6.7
1975	1,349	1,362	+0.3	326	+5.2	608	+3.4	428	-7.0
1976	1,337	1,358	-0.3	336	+3.1	632	+3.9	390	-8.9
1977	1,339	1,356	-0.1	344	+2.4	645	+2.1	367	-5.9
1978	1,340	1,358	+0.1	348	+1.2	666	+3.3	344	-6.3
1979	1,354	1,374	+1.2	363	+4.3	678	+1.8	333	-3.2
1980	1,360	1,385	+0.8	377	+3.9	697	+2.8	311	-6.6
1981	1,377	1,401	+1.2	383	+1.6	715	+2.6	303	-2.6
1982	1,406	1,432	+2.2	402	+5.0	742	+3.8	288	-5.0
1983	1,432	1,466	+2.4	421	+4.7	764	+3.0	281	-2.4
1984	1,445	1,477	+0.8	427	+1.4	777	+1.7	273	-2.8
1985	1,434	1,473	-0.2	441	+3.3	776	-0.1	256	-6.2
1986	1,426	1,469	-0.3	455	+3.2	776	-0.0	238	-7.0
1987	1,406	1,465	-0.3	467	+2.6	789	+1.7	209	-12.2
1988	1,391	1,442	-1.6	479	+2.6	792	+0.3	171	-18.7
1989	1,429	1,457	+1.0	488	+1.9	812	+2.5	157	-8.2
1990	1,412	1,470	+0.9	489	+0.2	829	+2.1	152	-3.2
1991	1,411	1,484	+1.0	501	+2.4	838	+1.1	145	-4.6
1992	1,404	1,484	+0.0	501	+0.0	848	+1.2	135	-6.9
1993	1,415[2]	1,493	+0.6	507	+1.2	857	+1.1	129	-4.4
1994	1,422	1,501	+0.5	509	+0.4	868	+1.3	124	-3.9

[1] Excludes American Samoa, Guam, Puerto Rico, and the Virgin Islands.
[2] Updated information.

Table 2
PUBLIC AND PRIVATE BASIC RN PROGRAMS, BY TYPE OF PROGRAM: 1985 TO 1994[1]

PUBLIC AND PRIVATE NURSING PROGRAMS	NUMBER OF PROGRAMS									
	1985	1986	1987	1988	1989	1990	1991	1992	1993	1994
All Programs	**1,473**	**1,469**	**1,465**	**1,442**	**1,457**	**1,470**	**1,484**	**1,484**	**1,493**	**1,501**
Public	942	950	970	979	1,005	1,020	1.038	1,036	1,048	1,056
Private	531	519	495	463	452	450	446	448	445	445
Baccalaureate	441	455	467	479	488	489	501	501	507	509
Public	217	227	235	239	245	248	254	254	260	265
Private	224	228	232	240	243	241	247	247	247	244
Associate Degree	776	776	789	792	812	829	838	848	857	868
Public	688	688	698	704	726	741	750	754	758	764
Private	88	88	91	88	86	88	88	94	99	104
Diploma	256	238	209	171	157	152	145	135	129	124
Public	37	35	37	36	34	31	34	28	30	27
Private	219	203	172	135	123	121	111	107	99	97

[1] Excludes American Samoa, Guam, Puerto Rico, and the Virgin Islands.

Table 3
ALL BASIC RN PROGRAMS, BY NLN REGION AND STATE: 1985 TO 1994[1]

NLN REGION AND STATE	NUMBER OF PROGRAMS									
	1985	1986	1987	1988	1989	1990	1991	1992	1993	1994
United States	**1,473**	**1,469**	**1,465**	**1,442**	**1,457**	**1,470**	**1,484**	**1,484**	**1,493**	**1,501**
North Atlantic	350	359	355	343	335	331	335	332	329	329
Midwest	433	429	424	415	423	429	430	429	435	434
South	485	478	481	475	483	489	497	500	507	513
West	205	203	205	209	216	221	222	223	222	225
Alabama	36	36	35	35	35	34	33	34	34	36
Alaska	2	2	2	2	3	2	2	2	2	2
Arizona	16	15	15	15	15	15	15	16	16	16
Arkansas	20	20	21	21	21	21	23	24	24	22
California	92	90	89	90	91	91	92	93	93	94
Colorado	14	13	12	12	12	17	17	17	17	17
Connecticut	18	18	18	18	18	18	19	17	17	17
Delaware	6	6	6	6	7	7	7	7	7	7
District of Columbia	6	6	6	5	5	5	5	5	5	5
Florida	39	40	40	40	40	39	39	40	40	40
Georgia	34	34	33	32	33	32	33	32	32	32
Hawaii	6	6	6	6	7	7	7	6	7	7
Idaho	6	6	7	7	7	7	7	7	7	7
Illinois	76	77	72	72	70	69	69	67	70	71
Indiana	37	36	40	42	44	46	44	46	46	46
Iowa	39	39	36	36	37	40	40	40	40	40
Kansas	30	30	32	33	32	32	32	30	30	30
Kentucky	28	28	27	27	29	32	32	33	34	34
Louisiana	22	22	22	21	21	23	23	21	22	23
Maine	10	14	15	15	14	14	14	14	15	15
Maryland	25	24	24	23	23	23	24	24	24	24
Massachusetts	47	46	48	44	41	42	43	42	42	43
Michigan	50	50	49	48	49	50	50	49	50	50
Minnesota	25	25	23	23	20	20	21	21	21	21
Mississippi	22	21	21	21	21	21	21	21	23	23
Missouri	41	41	42	40	44	45	47	46	47	46
Montana	4	6	4	4	5	5	5	5	5	5
Nebraska	14	13	13	10	13	15	13	13	13	13
Nevada	5	5	7	7	6	6	6	6	6	6
New Hampshire	11	10	10	10	9	9	9	9	9	9
New Jersey	39	38	38	38	38	39	38	38	37	37
New Mexico	12	13	13	14	14	14	14	14	14	16
New York	105	110	108	103	101	99	101	103	100	100
North Carolina	57	56	57	57	59	61	62	62	62	62
North Dakota	9	9	8	6	7	6	7	7	7	7
Ohio	70	69	70	67	68	67	68	69	70	69
Oklahoma	27	27	27	27	27	27	27	27	28	28
Oregon	17	17	17	18	18	18	18	18	16	16
Pennsylvania	98	98	94	92	90	87	88	86	86	84
Rhode Island	7	7	7	7	7	6	6	6	6	7
South Carolina	20	19	20	20	20	20	21	20	20	20
South Dakota	9	8	9	9	10	9	8	10	10	10
Tennessee	33	35	35	35	34	35	35	35	35	36
Texas	65	64	64	64	68	69	70	72	73	77
Utah	4	4	4	4	7	7	7	7	7	7
Vermont	5	5	5	5	5	5	5	5	5	5
Virginia	37	35	35	34	34	34	35	36	37	37
Washington	22	23	23	24	24	24	24	24	24	24
West Virginia	18	18	20	18	18	18	19	19	19	19
Wisconsin	33	32	30	29	29	30	31	31	31	31
Wyoming	5	5	6	6	7	8	8	8	8	8
American Samoa	1	1	1	1	1	1	1	1	1	1
Guam	1	1	1	1	1	1	1	1	1	1
Puerto Rico	20	20	20	22	22	22	25	28	29	31
Virgin Islands	2	2	2	2	2	2	2	2	2	2

[1] National and regional totals exclude American Samoa, Guam, Puerto Rico, and the Virgin Islands.

Table 4
BASIC BACCALAUREATE NURSING PROGRAMS, BY NLN REGION AND STATE: 1985 TO 1994[1]

NLN REGION AND STATE	NUMBER OF PROGRAMS									
	1985	1986	1987	1988	1989	1990	1991	1992	1993	1994
United States	**441**	**455**	**467**	**479**	**488**	**489**	**501**	**501**	**507**	**509**
North Atlantic	107	109	110	111	110	109	111	111	113	113
Midwest	131	139	144	151	157	157	161	159	161	160
South	151	154	158	162	165	165	170	172	175	177
West	52	53	55	55	56	58	59	59	58	59
Alabama	13	13	13	13	13	12	12	12	12	12
Alaska	1	1	1	1	1	1	1	1	1	1
Arizona	4	4	4	4	4	4	4	4	4	4
Arkansas	7	7	7	7	7	7	7	8	9	9
California	21	21	21	21	21	22	23	23	23	23
Colorado	5	6	6	6	6	7	7	7	7	7
Connecticut	7	7	7	7	7	7	7	7	8	8
Delaware	2	2	2	2	2	2	2	2	2	2
District of Columbia	5	5	5	4	4	4	4	4	4	4
Florida	12	13	13	13	13	13	13	13	13	13
Georgia	13	13	12	12	13	12	12	12	12	12
Hawaii	2	2	2	2	2	2	2	2	3	3
Idaho	1	1	2	2	2	2	2	2	2	2
Illinois	22	24	24	26	27	27	28	27	27	27
Indiana	13	13	17	20	21	21	21	21	21	20
Iowa	10	11	11	11	11	12	12	12	12	12
Kansas	10	10	11	11	10	10	10	10	11	11
Kentucky	8	9	9	9	10	10	10	10	10	10
Louisiana	12	12	12	12	12	12	12	12	13	13
Maine	3	3	5	6	6	6	6	6	7	7
Maryland	6	6	6	6	6	6	7	7	7	7
Massachusetts	14	14	15	14	14	14	15	15	15	15
Michigan	13	14	14	14	14	14	14	13	14	14
Minnesota	10	11	11	11	8	8	9	9	9	9
Mississippi	7	7	7	7	7	7	7	7	7	7
Missouri	11	11	11	11	14	14	15	15	15	15
Montana	2	2	2	2	2	2	2	2	2	2
Nebraska	7	7	7	7	7	7	6	6	6	6
Nevada	1	1	2	2	2	2	2	2	2	2
New Hampshire	3	3	3	3	3	3	3	3	3	3
New Jersey	7	7	7	7	7	7	7	7	7	7
New Mexico	1	1	1	1	1	1	1	1	1	2
New York	32	33	32	33	32	31	32	32	32	32
North Carolina	12	12	12	12	12	12	12	12	12	12
North Dakota	4	4	4	6	7	6	7	7	7	7
Ohio	15.	17	18	18	21	21	22	22	22	22
Oklahoma	11	11	11	11	11	11	11	11	11	11
Oregon	4	4	4	4	5	5	5	5	3	3
Pennsylvania	30	30	30	31	31	31	31	31	31	31
Rhode Island	3	3	3	3	3	3	3	3	3	3
South Carolina	6	6	6	7	7	7	7	7	7	7
South Dakota	3	3	3	3	4	4	4	4	4	4
Tennessee	9	11	12	14	14	15	16	16	16	17
Texas	21	20	20	21	22	23	24	25	25	26
Utah	3	3	3	3	3	3	3	3	3	3
Vermont	1	1	1	1	1	1	1	1	1	1
Virginia	9	9	10	10	10	10	11	11	12	12
Washington	6	6	6	6	6	6	6	6	6	6
West Virginia	5	6	8	8	8	8	9	9	9	9
Wisconsin	13	14	13	13	13	13	13	13	13	13
Wyoming	1	1	1	1	1	1	1	1	1	1
American Samoa	0	0	0	0	0	0	0	0	0	0
Guam	0	0	0	1	1	1	1	1	1	1
Puerto Rico	12	12	12	13	13	13	13	13	14	14
Virgin Islands	1	1	1	1	1	1	1	1	1	1

[1] National and regional totals exclude American Samoa, Guam, Puerto Rico, and the Virgin Islands.

Table 5
ASSOCIATE DEGREE NURSING PROGRAMS, BY NLN REGION AND STATE: 1985 TO 1994[1]

NLN REGION AND STATE	NUMBER OF PROGRAMS									
	1985	1986	1987	1988	1989	1990	1991	1992	1993	1994
United States	**776**	**776**	**789**	**792**	**812**	**829**	**838**	**848**	**857**	**868**
North Atlantic	137	144	147	146	148	147	151	152	151	153
Midwest	205	203	209	211	218	227	228	232	238	241
South	285	281	284	282	287	293	297	301	305	309
West	149	148	149	153	159	162	162	163	163	165
Alabama	20	20	20	20	20	20	20	21	21	23
Alaska	1	1	1	1	2	1	1	1	1	1
Arizona	12	11	11	11	11	11	11	12	12	12
Arkansas	11	11	12	12	12	12	14	14	13	11
California	69	68	67	68	69	68	68	69	69	70
Colorado	7	6	6	6	6	10	10	10	10	10
Connecticut	6	6	6	6	6	6	7	7	6	6
Delaware	3	3	3	3	4	4	4	4	4	4
District of Columbia	1	1	1	1	4	1	1	1	1	1
Florida	26	26	26	26	26	25	25	26	26	26
Georgia	19	19	19	19	19	19	20	20	20	20
Hawaii	4	4	4	4	5	5	5	4	4	4
Idaho	5	5	5	5	5	5	5	5	5	5
Illinois	34	34	34	35	35	35	35	35	38	39
Indiana	18	17	17	19	20	23	22	24	24	25
Iowa	20	20	20	20	21	23	23	23	23	23
Kansas	17	17	19	20	21	21	21	19	19	19
Kentucky	20	19	18	18	19	22	22	23	24	24
Louisiana	6	6	6	6	6	8	8	8	8	9
Maine	5	9	9	9	8	8	8	8	8	8
Maryland	14	14	14	14	14	14	14	14	14	14
Massachusetts	19	19	20	19	19	20	20	20	20	21
Michigan	32	32	32	31	32	33	33	33	33	33
Minnesota	12	12	12	12	12	12	12	12	12	12
Mississippi	14	14	14	14	14	14	14	14	16	16
Missouri	20	20	22	21	22	23	24	25	26	27
Montana	2	2	2	2	3	3	3	3	3	3
Nebraska	2	1	1	2	5	7	6	6	6	6
Nevada	4	4	5	5	4	4	4	4	4	4
New Hampshire	6	6	6	6	6	6	6	6	6	6
New Jersey	14	13	14	14	14	15	14	14	14	14
New Mexico	11	12	12	13	13	13	13	13	13	14
New York	55	59	60	59	60	59	61	63	63	63
North Carolina	40	39	41	41	43	45	46	46	46	46
North Dakota	2	2	2	0	0	0	0	0	0	0
Ohio	29.	29	30	31	30	30	31	32	34	34
Oklahoma	16	16	16	16	16	16	16	16	17	17
Oregon	13	13	13	14	13	13	13	13	13	13
Pennsylvania	22	22	22	23	24	22	24	23	23	23
Rhode Island	2	2	2	2	2	2	2	2	2	3
South Carolina	13	12	13	13	13	13	14	13	13	13
South Dakota	4	4	5	5	5	4	4	6	6	6
Tennessee	17	17	17	17	16	16	15	15	15	15
Texas	42	42	42	41	44	44	44	45	46	49
Utah	1	1	1	1	4	4	4	4	4	4
Vermont	4	4	4	4	4	4	4	4	4	4
Virginia	16	16	16	16	16	16	16	17	17	17
Washington	16	17	17	18	18	18	18	18	18	18
West Virginia	11	10	10	9	9	9	9	9	9	9
Wisconsin	15	15	15	15	15	16	17	17	17	17
Wyoming	4	4	5	5	6	7	7	7	7	7
American Samoa	1	1	1	1	1	1	1	1	1	1
Guam	1	1	1	0	0	0	0	0	0	0
Puerto Rico	8	8	8	9	9	9	12	15	15	17
Virgin Islands	1	1	1	1	1	1	1	1	1	1

[1] National and regional totals exclude American Samoa, Guam, Puerto Rico, and the Virgin Islands.

Table 6
DIPLOMA NURSING PROGRAMS, BY NLN REGION AND STATE: 1985 TO 1994[1]

NLN REGION AND STATE	NUMBER OF PROGRAMS									
	1985	1986	1987	1988	1989	1990	1991	1992	1993	1994
United States	**256**	**238**	**209**	**171**	**157**	**152**	**145**	**135**	**129**	**124**
North Atlantic	106	106	98	86	77	75	73	69	65	63
Midwest	97	87	71	53	48	45	41	38	36	33
South	49	43	39	31	31	31	30	27	27	27
West	4	2	1	1	1	1	1	1	1	1
Alabama	3	3	2	2	2	2	1	1	1	1
Alaska	0	0	0	0	0	0	0	0	0	0
Arizona	0	0	0	0	0	0	0	0	0	0
Arkansas	2	2	2	2	2	2	2	2	2	2
California	2	1	1	1	1	1	1	1	1	1
Colorado	2	1	0	0	0	0	0	0	0	0
Connecticut	5	5	5	5	5	5	5	3	3	3
Delaware	1	1	1	1	1	1	1	1	1	1
District of Columbia	0	0	0	0	0	0	0	0	0	0
Florida	1	1	1	1	1	1	1	1	1	1
Georgia	2	2	2	1	1	1	1	0	0	0
Hawaii	0	0	0	0	0	0	0	0	0	0
Idaho	0	0	0	0	0	0	0	0	0	0
Illinois	20	19	14	11	8	7	6	5	5	5
Indiana	6	6	6	3	3	2	1	1	1	1
Iowa	9	8	5	5	5	5	5	5	5	5
Kansas	3	3	2	2	1	1	1	1	0	0
Kentucky	0	0	0	0	0	0	0	0	0	0
Louisiana	4	4	4	3	3	3	3	1	1	1
Maine	2	2	1	0	0	0	0	0	0	0
Maryland	5	4	4	3	3	3	3	3	3	3
Massachusetts	14	13	13	11	8	8	8	7	7	7
Michigan	5	4	3	3	3	3	3	3	3	3
Minnesota	3	2	0	0	0	0	0	0	0	0
Mississippi	1	0	0	0	0	0	0	0	0	0
Missouri	10	10	9	8	8	8	8	6	6	4
Montana	0	0	0	0	0	0	0	0	0	0
Nebraska	5	5	5	1	1	1	1	1	1	1
Nevada	0	0	0	0	0	0	0	0	0	0
New Hampshire	2	1	1	1	0	0	0	0	0	0
New Jersey	18	18	17	17	17	17	17	17	16	16
New Mexico	0	0	0	0	0	0	0	0	0	0
New York	18	18	16	11	9	9	8	8	5	5
North Carolina	5	5	4	4	4	4	4	4	4	4
North Dakota	3	3	2	0	0	0	0	0	0	0
Ohio	26.	23	22	18	17	16	15	15	14	13
Oklahoma	0	0	0	0	0	0	0	0	0	0
Oregon	0	0	0	0	0	0	0	0	0	0
Pennsylvania	46	46	42	38	35	34	33	32	32	30
Rhode Island	2	2	2	2	2	1	1	1	1	1
South Carolina	1	1	1	0	0	0	0	0	0	0
South Dakota	2	1	1	1	1	1	0	0	0	0
Tennessee	7	7	6	4	4	4	4	4	4	4
Texas	2	2	2	2	2	2	2	2	2	2
Utah	0	0	0	0	0	0	0	0	0	0
Vermont	0	0	0	0	0	0	0	0	0	0
Virginia	12	10	9	8	8	8	8	8	8	8
Washington	0	0	0	0	0	0	0	0	0	0
West Virginia	2	2	2	1	1	1	1	1	1	1
Wisconsin	5	3	2	1	1	1	1	1	1	1
Wyoming	0	0	0	0	0	0	0	0	0	0
American Samoa	0	0	0	0	0	0	0	0	0	0
Guam	0	0	0	0	0	0	0	0	0	0
Puerto Rico	0	0	0	0	0	0	0	0	0	0
Virgin Islands	0	0	0	0	0	0	0	0	0	0

[1] National and regional totals exclude American Samoa, Guam, Puerto Rico, and the Virgin Islands.

Table 7
BACCALAUREATE NURSING PROGRAMS THAT ENROLL BASIC AND/OR RN STUDENTS, BY NLN ACCREDITATION STATUS: JANUARY, 1995[1]

NLN ACCREDITATION STATUS	TOTAL NUMBER OF PROGRAMS	TYPE OF STUDENT ENROLLED	
		Both Basic and RN Students	RN Students Only
Total	**646**	**509**	**137**
Accredited	600	483	117
Non-Accredited	46	26	20

[1] Excludes American Samoa, Guam, Puerto Rico, and the Virgin Islands.

Table 8
BASIC RN PROGRAMS, BY TYPE OF PROGRAM AND NLN ACCREDITATION STATUS: JANUARY, 1995[1]

NLN REGION AND STATE	ALL BASIC RN PROGRAMS			BACCALAUREATE PROGRAMS			ASSOCIATE DEGREE PROGRAMS			DIPLOMA PROGRAMS		
	Total	Accredited	Not Accredited	Total	Accredited	Not Accredited	Total	Accredited	Not Accredited	Total	Accredited	Not Accredited
United States	**1,501**	**1,202**	**299**	**509**	**483**	**26**	**868**	**595**	**273**	**124**	**124**	**0**
North Atlantic	329	298	31	113	112	1	153	123	30	63	63	0
Midwest	434	335	99	160	149	11	241	153	88	33	33	0
South	513	409	104	177	165	12	309	217	92	27	27	0
West	225	160	65	59	57	2	165	102	63	1	1	0
Alabama	36	31	5	12	12	0	23	18	5	1	1	0
Alaska	2	2	0	1	1	0	1	1	0	0	0	0
Arizona	16	14	2	4	4	0	12	10	2	0	0	0
Arkansas	22	20	2	9	8	1	11	10	1	2	2	0
California	94	52	42	23	23	0	70	28	42	1	1	0
Colorado	17	10	7	7	6	1	10	4	6	0	0	0
Connecticut	17	16	1	8	7	1	6	6	0	3	3	0
Delaware	7	5	2	2	2	0	4	2	2	1	1	0
District of Columbia	5	5	0	4	4	0	1	1	0	0	0	0
Florida	40	27	13	13	11	2	26	15	11	1	1	0
Georgia	32	31	1	12	11	1	20	20	0	0	0	0
Hawaii	7	5	2	3	2	1	4	3	1	0	0	0
Idaho	7	7	0	2	2	0	5	5	0	0	0	0
Illinois	71	48	23	27	22	5	39	21	18	5	5	0
Indiana	46	40	6	20	20	0	25	19	6	1	1	0
Iowa	40	22	18	12	11	1	23	6	17	5	5	0
Kansas	30	29	1	11	10	1	19	19	0	0	0	0
Kentucky	34	26	8	10	10	0	24	16	8	0	0	0
Louisiana	23	20	3	13	13	0	9	6	3	1	1	0
Maine	15	15	0	7	7	0	8	8	0	0	0	0
Maryland	24	18	6	7	6	1	14	9	5	3	3	0
Massachusetts	43	41	2	15	15	0	21	19	2	7	7	0
Michigan	50	26	24	14	13	1	33	10	23	3	3	0
Minnesota	21	17	4	9	9	0	12	8	4	0	0	0
Mississippi	23	21	2	7	7	0	16	14	2	0	0	0
Missouri	46	32	14	15	14	1	27	14	13	4	4	0
Montana	5	5	0	2	2	0	3	3	0	0	0	0
Nebraska	13	12	1	6	6	0	6	5	1	1	1	0
Nevada	6	6	0	2	2	0	4	4	0	0	0	0
New Hampshire	9	6	3	3	3	0	6	3	3	0	0	0
New Jersey	37	37	0	7	7	0	14	14	0	16	16	0
New Mexico	16	13	3	2	2	0	14	11	3	0	0	0
New York	100	81	19	32	32	0	63	44	19	5	5	0
North Carolina	62	25	37	12	12	0	46	9	37	4	4	0
North Dakota	7	7	0	7	7	0	0	0	0	0	0	0
Ohio	69	63	6	22	20	2	34	30	4	13	13	0
Oklahoma	28	27	1	11	11	0	17	16	1	0	0	0
Oregon	16	11	5	3	3	0	13	8	5	0	0	0
Pennsylvania	84	81	3	31	31	0	23	20	3	30	30	0
Rhode Island	7	6	1	3	3	0	3	2	1	1	1	0
South Carolina	20	15	5	7	6	1	13	9	4	0	0	0
South Dakota	10	8	2	4	4	0	6	4	2	0	0	0
Tennessee	36	34	2	17	15	2	15	15	0	4	4	0
Texas	77	60	17	26	23	3	49	35	14	2	2	0
Utah	7	7	0	3	3	0	4	4	0	0	0	0
Vermont	5	5	0	1	1	0	4	4	0	0	0	0
Virginia	37	36	1	12	12	0	17	16	1	8	8	0
Washington	24	20	4	6	6	0	18	14	4	0	0	0
West Virginia	19	18	1	9	8	1	9	9	0	1	1	0
Wisconsin	31	31	0	13	13	0	17	17	0	1	1	0
Wyoming	8	8	0	1	1	0	7	7	0	0	0	0
American Samoa	1	0	1	0	0	0	1	0	1	0	0	0
Guam	1	0	1	1	0	1	0	0	0	0	0	0
Puerto Rico	31	13	18	14	7	7	17	6	11	0	0	0
Virgin Islands	2	2	0	1	1	0	1	1	0	0	0	0

[1] National and regional totals exclude American Samoa, Guam, Puerto Rico, and the Virgin Islands.

Table 9
MEAN ANNUAL TUITIONS OF FULL-TIME STUDENTS IN PUBLIC OR PRIVATE
BASIC RN PROGRAMS: 1994 TO 1995[1]

NURSING PROGRAMS	PRINCIPAL FINANCIAL SUPPORT OF SCHOOL		
	Public		Private
	Resident	Non-Resident	
All Programs	$1,762	$4,399	$7,965
Basic Baccalaureate	$2,364	$6,081	$9,941
Associate Degree	$1,480	$3,768	$7,011
Diploma	$4,247	$4,167	$4,266

[1] Excludes American Samoa, Guam, Puerto Rico, and the Virgin Islands.

Table 10
FALL ADMISSIONS TO PUBLIC AND PRIVATE BASIC RN PROGRAMS, BY TYPE OF PROGRAM: 1985 TO 1994[1]

PUBLIC AND PRIVATE NURSING PROGRAMS	NUMBER OF FALL ADMISSIONS									
	1985	1986	1987	1988	1989	1990	1991	1992	1993	1994
All Programs	**83,026**	**70,581**	**68,745**	**74,921**	**79,570**	**86,125**	**90,499**	**96,786**	**96,864**	**96,107**
Public	57,018	50,417	51,362	56,922	60,032	64,410	67,163	70,106	70,216	69,761
Private	26,008	20,164	17,383	17,999	19,538	21,715	23,336	26,680	26,648	26,346
Baccalaureate	28,883	23,765	19,985	20,749	21,544	25,117	27,361	31,719	32,403	33,124
Public	16,239	13,356	12,806	13,122	13,574	15,648	16,369	18,064	18,542	18,422
Private	12,644	10,409	7,179	7,627	7,970	9,469	10,992	13,655	13,861	14,702
Associate Degree	44,966	40,166	41,695	46,910	49,930	52,674	54,732	56,828	56,514	56,035
Public	39,617	36,070	37,389	42,357	44,840	47,175	49,124	50,777	50,170	50,200
Private	5,349	4,096	4,306	4,553	5,090	5,499	5,608	6,051	6,344	5,835
Diploma	9,177	6,650	7,065	7,262	8,096	8,334	8,406	8,239	7,947	6,948
Public	1,162	991	1,167	1,443	1,618	1,587	1,670	1,265	1,504	1,139
Private	8,015	5,659	5,898	5,819	6,478	6,747	6,736	6,974	6,443	5,809

[1] Excludes American Samoa, Guam, Puerto Rico, and the Virgin Islands.

Table 11
ANNUAL ADMISSIONS TO BASIC RN PROGRAMS AND PERCENTAGE CHANGE FROM PREVIOUS YEAR, BY TYPE OF PROGRAM: 1974-75 TO 1993-94[1]

ACADEMIC YEAR	ALL BASIC RN PROGRAMS		BACCALAUREATE PROGRAMS		ASSOCIATE DEGREE PROGRAMS		DIPLOMA PROGRAMS	
	Number of Admissions	Percent Change	Number of Admissions	Percent Change	Number of Admissions	Percent Change	Number of Admissions	Percent Change
1974-75	109,020	+1.6	34,956	+7.7	49,368	+3.0	24,696	-8.3
1975-76	112,174	+2.9	36,320	+3.9	52,232	+5.8	23,622	-4.3
1976-77	112,523	+0.3	36,670	+1.0	53,610	+2.6	22,243	-5.8
1977-78	110,950	-1.4	37,348	+1.8	52,991	-1.1	20,611	-7.3
1978-79	107,476	-3.2	35,611	-4.7	53,366	+0.7	18,499	-10.2
1979-80	105,952	-1.4	35,414	-0.5	53,633	+0.5	16,905	-8.6
1980-81	110,201	+4.0	35,808	+1.1	56,899	+6.1	17,494	+3.5
1981-82	115,279	+4.6	35,928	+0.3	60,423	+6.1	18,928	+8.1
1982-83	120,579	+4.6	37,264	+3.7	63,947	+5.8	19,368	+2.3
1983-84	123,824	+2.7	39,400	+5.7	66,576	+4.1	17,848	-7.8
1984-85	118,224	-4.5	39,573	+0.4	63,776	-4.2	14,875	-16.7
1985-86	100,791	-14.7	34,310	-13.3	56,635	-11.2	9,846	-33.0
1986-87	90,693	-10.0	28,026	-18.3	54,330	-4.1	8,337	-15.3
1987-88	94,269	+3.9	28,505	+1.7	57,375	+5.6	8,389	+0.6
1988-89	103,025	+9.3	29,042	+1.9	63,973	+11.5	10,010	+19.3
1989-90	108,580	+5.4	29,858	+2.6	68,634	+7.3	10,088	+0.8
1990-91	113,526	+4.6	33,437	+12.0	69,869	+1.8	10,220	-1.3
1991-92	122,656	+8.0	37,886	+13.3	74,079	+6.0	10,691	+4.6
1992-93	126,837	+3.4	41,290	+9.0	75,382	+1.7	10,165	-4.9
1993-94	129,897	+2.4	42,953	+4.0	77,343	+2.6	9,601	-5.5

[1] Excludes American Samoa, Guam, Puerto Rico, and the Virgin Islands.

Table 12
ANNUAL ADMISSIONS TO PUBLIC AND PRIVATE BASIC RN PROGRAMS, BY TYPE OF PROGRAM: 1984-85 TO 1993-94[1]

PUBLIC AND PRIVATE NURSING PROGRAMS	NUMBER OF ANNUAL ADMISSIONS									
	1984-85	1985-86	1986-87	1987-88	1988-89	1989-90	1990-91	1991-92	1992-93	1993-94
All Programs	**118,224**	**100,791**	**90,693**	**94,269**	**103,025**	**108,580**	**113,526**	**122,656**	**126,837**	**129,897**
Public	81,198	71,921	67,890	71,866	77,892	82,686	88,764	92,720	94,572	96,296
Private	37,026	28,870	22,803	22,403	25,133	25,894	24,762	29,936	32,265	33,601
Baccalaureate	39,573	34,310	28,026	28,505	29,042	29,858	33,437	37,886	41,290	42,953
Public	23,871	19,747	18,057	18,622	18,824	19,492	22,252	23,484	24,345	24,861
Private	15,702	14,563	9,969	9,883	10,218	10,366	11,185	14,402	16,945	18,092
Associate Degree	63,776	56,635	54,330	57,375	63,973	68,634	69,869	74,079	75,382	77,343
Public	55,150	50,549	48,249	51,566	56,958	61,151	64,258	67,146	68,075	69,562
Private	8,626	6,086	6,081	5,809	7,015	7,483	5,611	6,933	7,307	7,781
Diploma	14,875	9,846	8,337	8,389	10,010	10,088	10,220	10,691	10,165	9,601
Public	2,177	1,625	1,584	1,678	2,110	2,043	2,254	2,090	2,152	1,873
Private	12,698	8,221	6,753	6,711	7,900	8,045	7,966	8,601	8,013	7,728

1 Excludes American Samoa, Guam, Puerto Rico, and the Virgin Islands.

Table 13
ANNUAL ADMISSIONS TO ALL BASIC RN PROGRAMS, BY NLN REGION AND STATE: 1984-85 TO 1993-94[1]

NLN REGION AND STATE	NUMBER OF ADMISSIONS									
	1984-85	1985-86	1986-87	1987-88	1988-89	1989-90	1990-91	1991-92	1992-93	1993-94
United States	**118,224**	**100,791**	**90,693**	**94,269**	**103,025**	**108,580**	**113,526**	**122,656**	**126,837**	**129,897**
North Atlantic	31,738	27,818	23,069	23,792	25,876	26,889	27,349	30,556	32,589	33,140
Midwest	33,478	27,305	25,151	24,647	26,862	28,410	29,602	32,527	33,579	34,840
South	38,089	31,702	29,632	32,380	36,083	39,397	42,468	45,062	45,764	46,979
West	14,919	13,966	12,841	13,450	14,204	13,884	14,107	14,511	14,905	14,938
Alabama	3,074	2,158	2,149	2,003	2,346	2,574	2,570	3,108	3,488	3,847
Alaska	188	171	166	166	266	81	103	102	105	110
Arizona	1,213	1,024	962	970	996	929	1,110	1,196	1,237	1,281
Arkansas	1,143	937	983	1,327	1,415	1,545	1,723	1,821	1,802	1,751
California	7,568	7,013	6,098	6,320	6,507	6,340	6,465	6,577	6,691	6,710
Colorado	854	787	942	873	1,092	926	1,011	1,020	1,064	1,041
Connecticut	1,372	1,266	1,012	1,200	1,200	1,070	1,141	1,513	1,370	1,049
Delaware	416	413	339	370	386	394	316	455	580	532
District of Columbia	628	627	334	449	315	248	361	327	555	355
Florida	4,269	3,508	3,426	3,651	3,849	4,400	4,551	4,688	4,930	4,835
Georgia	2,953	2,060	1,805	2,075	2,289	2,725	2,566	3,003	3,252	3,366
Hawaii	262	372	183	345	272	361	281	301	409	395
Idaho	298	303	274	391	332	338	372	331	333	352
Illinois	5,881	5,255	4,422	3,840	4,642	4,453	4,889	5,284	5,317	5,774
Indiana	3,055	2,551	2,480	2,496	2,581	2,594	2,820	3,038	3,213	3,257
Iowa	2,206	1,625	1,661	1,668	1,672	1,852	1,938	2,146	2,418	2,358
Kansas	1,571	1,131	957	1,165	1,244	1,613	1,521	1,610	1,831	1,603
Kentucky	2,180	2,236	1,683	1,879	2,093	2,159	3,048	2,729	2,676	2,757
Louisiana	2,062	1,768	1,432	1,558	1,741	2,081	3,100	2,970	2,813	3,156
Maine	650	490	433	421	514	498	579	490	797	602
Maryland	2,313	1,788	1,483	1,449	1,542	1,566	1,819	2,166	2,268	2,269
Massachusetts	3,558	3,065	2,700	2,545	2,536	3,082	3,020	3,415	3,422	3,386
Michigan	4,820	3,893	3,872	3,521	3,582	3,748	3,890	4,308	4,139	4,236
Minnesota	1,779	1,343	1,431	1,570	1,788	1,939	1,759	1,974	2,042	1,997
Mississippi	1,825	1,524	1,503	1,440	1,584	1,988	2,089	2,144	2,184	2,211
Missouri	2,430	2,081	2,087	1,962	2,196	2,350	2,535	3,049	2,999	3,380
Montana	312	305	284	322	347	334	366	368	355	387
Nebraska	1,366	567	749	663	845	978	859	891	960	1,051
Nevada	251	204	199	268	215	256	281	268	283	319
New Hampshire	523	412	372	422	360	538	504	551	579	543
New Jersey	4,016	3,275	2,521	2,890	3,198	2,913	3,426	3,794	3,574	3,631
New Mexico	552	421	455	731	713	788	778	798	710	824
New York	12,601	11,845	9,401	9,122	10,638	10,861	10,735	11,678	12,571	13,942
North Carolina	3,007	2,796	2,920	2,881	3,526	3,753	3,599	3,597	3,833	4,141
North Dakot	609	327	225	191	301	374	341	381	320	406
Ohio	6,302	5,203	4,767	4,960	5,386	5,824	6,086	6,232	6,771	7,374
Oklahoma	1,182	1,232	1,244	1,335	1,350	1,513	1,642	1,761	1,657	1,710
Oregon	1,031	924	953	875	963	975	968	1,017	981	938
Pennsylvania	6,739	5,742	5,335	5,758	6,100	6,564	6,421	7,136	7,934	8,142
Rhode Island	962	522	440	402	382	486	579	886	902	673
South Carolina	1,587	1,231	1,031	1,239	1,387	1,579	1,763	1,742	1,673	1,778
South Dakota	628	361	629	542	365	486	473	561	579	554
Tennessee	3,099	2,341	2,179	2,848	2,702	3,025	2,940	3,191	3,440	3,654
Texas	5,514	5,053	4,758	5,631	6,880	6,905	7,273	7,851	7,533	7,344
Utah	447	473	345	450	507	810	523	680	719	685
Vermont	273	211	182	213	247	235	267	311	305	285
Virginia	2,588	2,024	2,035	2,149	2,597	2,551	2,665	3,151	3,030	3,027
Washington	1,730	1,751	1,769	1,544	1,770	1,547	1,552	1,527	1,704	1,626
West Virginia	1,293	1,046	1,001	915	1,052	1,033	1,120	1,140	1,185	1,133
Wisconsin	2,831	2,968	1,871	2,069	2,278	2,199	2,491	3,053	2,990	2,850
Wyoming	195	168	211	195	224	199	297	326	314	270
American Samoa	0	34	11	11	11	11	10	11	12	12
Guam	19	29	29	0	25	20	25	25	19	20
Puerto Rico	2,134	3,263	3,048	1,945	1,729	1,816	1,507	1,398	1,859	1,570
Virgin Islands	26	28	36	19	12	19	20	27	40	65

[1] National and regional totals exclude American Samoa, Guam, Puerto Rico, and the Virgin Islands.

Table 14
ANNUAL ADMISSIONS TO BASIC BACCALAUREATE NURSING PROGRAMS, BY NLN REGION AND STATE: 1984-85 TO 1993-94[1]

NLN REGION AND STATE	NUMBER OF ADMISSIONS									
	1984-85	1985-86	1986-87	1987-88	1988-89	1989-90	1990-91	1991-92	1992-93	1993-94
United States	**39,573**	**34,310**	**28,026**	**28,505**	**29,042**	**29,858**	**33,437**	**37,886**	**41,290**	**42,953**
North Atlantic	10,987	9,491	6,545	6,449	6,525	6,412	6,549	7,612	9,845	9,746
Midwest	10,846	9,704	8,394	8,267	8,439	8,614	9,258	11,380	12,391	13,154
South	12,866	10,584	9,064	9,666	9,937	11,145	13,240	14,419	14,475	15,299
West	4,874	4,531	4,023	4,123	4,141	3,687	4,390	4,475	4,579	4,754
Alabama	1,367	861	976	834	853	915	821	1,096	1,086	1,091
Alaska	126	132	126	126	226	38	53	65	69	78
Arizona	455	314	279	270	287	191	270	285	337	347
Arkansas	313	258	289	310	321	317	447	426	471	591
California	2,142	2,083	1,746	1,720	1,595	1,371	1,769	1,802	1,696	1,768
Colorado	361	347	398	299	455	350	460	409	477	506
Connecticut	520	374	349	516	574	277	342	656	707	456
Delaware	209	171	117	117	122	88	72	188	278	256
District of Columbia	508	562	255	359	225	199	279	263	491	293
Florida	994	926	714	652	770	779	915	925	1,015	940
Georgia	925	725	503	561	769	987	755	940	909	1,016
Hawaii	115	147	119	170	59	152	104	101	185	196
Idaho	45	45	44	78	87	69	85	74	90	90
Illinois	1,603	1,694	1,354	1,162	1,242	1,052	1,341	1,645	1,851	2,278
Indiana	1,224	1,207	1,082	1,116	1,092	995	1,188	1,271	1,362	1,338
Iowa	596	451	394	377	354	436	367	467	542	489
Kansas	520	436	353	403	428	523	507	643	899	694
Kentucky	612	977	554	607	662	566	815	738	635	785
Louisiana	996	974	790	911	1,009	1,247	2,184	1,925	1,708	2,086
Maine	329	206	205	226	311	283	338	196	426	237
Maryland	772	612	466	388	306	377	554	740	829	762
Massachusetts	1,388	1,114	823	715	785	1,134	998	1,180	1,190	1,227
Michigan	1,301	1,100	1,177	1,069	1,080	968	1,137	1,232	1,298	1,344
Minnesota	549	503	437	445	418	503	475	568	769	688
Mississippi	638	407	362	322	348	570	689	738	665	684
Missouri	650	631	569	601	557	528	702	1,019	967	1,262
Montana	199	187	176	220	187	221	239	233	224	258
Nebraska	721	346	608	538	610	648	499	572	617	745
Nevada	61	42	43	71	75	85	118	90	126	114
New Hampshire	161	117	110	81	99	136	151	168	175	162
New Jersey	1,168	1,027	528	681	408	386	397	459	422	562
New Mexico	96	26	55	77	74	145	227	192	40	128
New York	3,627	3,669	2,339	1,957	2,115	1,948	1,759	1,765	2,613	2,948
North Carolina	779	587	837	553	587	658	808	814	1,038	1,122
North Dakota	331	179	162	191	301	374	341	381	320	406
Ohio	1,820	1,389	1,265	1,219	1,282	1,507	1,447	1,916	2,077	2,272
Oklahoma	428	455	372	407	414	447	503	647	536	582
Oregon	359	292	370	288	286	327	369	434	378	376
Pennsylvania	2,329	2,025	1,611	1,618	1,738	1,724	1,931	2,080	2,903	3,259
Rhode Island	646	203	152	104	92	174	204	565	561	266
South Carolina	778	469	282	355	342	326	555	534	527	525
South Dakota	255	143	140	181	125	206	254	281	218	214
Tennessee	1,081	629	576	1,000	729	908	736	932	1,187	1,213
Texas	2,029	1,698	1,517	1,728	1,732	2,072	2,340	2,832	2,404	2,487
Utah	201	212	170	231	203	341	221	270	250	258
Vermont	102	73	56	75	56	63	78	92	79	80
Virginia	856	662	587	753	776	701	789	775	1,037	995
Washington	641	601	419	514	558	397	420	461	643	571
West Virginia	299	344	239	285	319	275	329	357	428	420
Wisconsin	1,276	1,625	853	965	950	874	1,000	1,385	1,471	1,424
Wyoming	73	53	78	59	49	0	55	59	64	64
American Samoa	0	0	0	—	—	—	—	0	0	0
Guam	0	0	0	0	25	20	25	25	19	20
Puerto Rico	1,587	2,466	2,335	1,301	996	900	672	686	786	804
Virgin Islands	10	10	18	9	7	5	10	18	25	42

[1] National and regional totals exclude American Samoa, Guam, Puerto Rico, and the Virgin Islands.

Table 15
ANNUAL ADMISSIONS TO ASSOCIATE DEGREE NURSING PROGRAMS, BY NLN REGION AND STATE: 1984-85 TO 1993-94[1]

NLN REGION AND STATE	NUMBER OF ANNUAL ADMISSIONS									
	1984-85	1985-86	1986-87	1987-88	1988-89	1989-90	1990-91	1991-92	1992-93	1993-94
United States	**63,776**	**56,635**	**54,330**	**57,375**	**63,973**	**68,634**	**69,869**	**74,079**	**75,382**	**77,343**
North Atlantic	14,889	14,089	12,800	13,592	14,792	15,970	15,952	17,990	18,018	18,893
Midwest	16,807	14,012	13,974	13,927	15,652	16,888	17,503	18,117	18,369	19,356
South	22,307	19,285	18,894	20,695	23,753	25,816	26,940	28,170	28,864	29,071
West	9,773	9,249	8,662	9,161	9,776	9,960	9,474	9,802	10,131	10,023
Alabama	1,584	1,265	1,139	1,136	1,457	1,632	1,719	1,956	2,348	2,710
Alaska	62	39	40	40	40	43	50	37	36	32
Arizona	776	710	683	700	709	738	840	911	900	934
Arkansas	661	576	543	705	767	870	861	954	911	795
California	5,196	4,744	4,196	4,434	4,625	4,732	4,453	4,541	4,800	4,781
Colorado	451	440	544	574	637	576	551	611	587	535
Connecticut	535	712	442	457	356	472	512	672	478	413
Delaware	187	224	205	236	245	276	212	237	272	248
District of Columbia	120	65	79	90	90	49	82	64	64	62
Florida	3,144	2,513	2,636	2,920	2,980	3,508	3,522	3,656	3,817	3,798
Georgia	1,890	1,233	1,215	1,420	1,432	1,738	1,811	2,063	2,343	2,350
Hawaii	147	225	64	175	213	209	177	200	224	199
Idaho	253	258	230	313	245	269	287	257	243	262
Illinois	3,142	2,847	2,723	2,418	3,024	3,032	3,247	3,342	3,139	3,244
Indiana	1,365	1,041	1,076	1,263	1,389	1,550	1,576	1,689	1,778	1,849
Iowa	1,246	968	1,006	1,124	1,111	1,114	1,237	1,293	1,466	1,582
Kansas	885	608	580	733	792	1,062	984	967	932	909
Kentucky	1,568	1,259	1,129	1,272	1,431	1,593	2,233	1,991	2,041	1,972
Louisiana	713	457	438	412	509	618	868	1,003	1,060	1,014
Maine	238	260	228	195	203	215	241	294	371	365
Maryland	1,226	1,077	899	927	1,079	1,061	1,098	1,220	1,235	1,324
Massachusetts	1,570	1,517	1,479	1,482	1,361	1,492	1,508	1,706	1,680	1,634
Michigan	3,155	2,489	2,451	2,298	2,348	2,584	2,458	2,763	2,586	2,647
Minnesota	1,133	840	994	1,125	1,370	1,436	1,284	1,406	1,273	1,309
Mississippi	1,187	1,117	1,141	1,118	1,236	1,418	1,400	1,406	1,519	1,527
Missouri	1,022	938	1,032	860	1,025	1,149	1,208	1,367	1,530	1,658
Montana	113	118	108	102	160	113	127	135	131	129
Nebraska	265	70	83	71	184	267	285	254	258	248
Nevada	190	162	156	197	140	171	163	178	157	205
New Hampshire	316	251	248	341	261	402	353	383	404	381
New Jersey	1,538	1,267	1,156	1,340	1,415	1,477	1,737	1,752	1,775	1,652
New Mexico	456	395	400	654	639	643	551	606	670	696
New York	8,036	7,521	6,592	6,743	8,013	8,453	8,494	9,496	9,643	10,761
North Carolina	1,960	2,042	1,969	2,150	2,414	2,741	2,501	2,499	2,513	2,666
North Dakota	156	89	63	—	—	—	—	—	—	—
Ohio	2,908	2,689	2,608	2,705	2,968	3,177	3,611	3,237	3,597	4,214
Oklahoma	754	777	872	928	936	1,066	1,139	1,114	1,121	1,128
Oregon	672	632	583	587	677	648	599	583	603	562
Pennsylvania	1,938	1,884	1,998	2,309	2,398	2,682	2,294	2,886	2,805	2,813
Rhode Island	240	250	247	261	259	280	330	281	300	359
South Carolina	803	749	740	884	1,045	1,253	1,208	1,208	1,146	1,253
South Dakota	289	186	385	305	217	280	219	280	361	340
Tennessee	1,266	1,261	1,301	1,432	1,462	1,630	1,767	1,771	1,675	1,649
Texas	3,341	3,245	3,111	3,764	4,948	4,641	4,725	4,779	4,898	4,625
Utah	246	267	175	219	304	469	302	410	469	427
Vermont	171	138	126	138	191	172	189	219	226	205
Virginia	1,325	1,073	1,150	1,077	1,406	1,374	1,377	1,854	1,566	1,625
Washington	1,089	1,150	1,350	1,030	1212	1,150	1,132	1,066	1,061	1,055
West Virginia	885	641	611	550	651	673	711	696	671	635
Wisconsin	1,241	1,247	973	1,025	1,224	1,237	1,394	1,519	1,449	1,356
Wyoming	122	115	133	136	175	199	242	267	250	206
American Samoa	0	34	11	11	11	11	10	11	12	12
Guam	29	29	29	—	—	—	—	—	—	—
Puerto Rico	547	797	713	644	733	916	835	712	1,073	766
Virgin Islands	216	18	18	10	5	14	10	9	15	23

[1] National and regional totals exclude American Samoa, Guam, Puerto Rico, and the Virgin Islands.

Table 16
ANNUAL ADMISSIONS TO DIPLOMA NURSING PROGRAMS, BY NLN REGION AND STATE: 1984-85 TO 1993-94[1]

NLN REGION AND STATE	NUMBER OF ANNUAL ADMISSIONS									
	1984-85	1985-86	1986-87	1987-88	1988-89	1989-90	1990-91	1991-92	1992-93	1993-94
United States	**14,875**	**9,846**	**8,337**	**8,389**	**10,010**	**10,088**	**10,220**	**10,691**	**10,165**	**9,601**
North Atlantic	5,862	4,238	3,724	3,751	4,559	4,507	4,848	4,954	4,726	4,501
Midwest	5,825	3,589	2,783	2,453	2,771	2,908	2,841	3,030	2,819	2,330
South	2,916	1,833	1,674	2,019	2,393	2,436	2,288	2,473	2,425	2,609
West	272	186	156	166	287	237	243	234	195	161
Alabama	123	32	34	33	36	27	30	56	54	46
Alaska	0	0	0	—	—	—	—	—	—	—
Arizona	0	0	0	—	—	—	—	—	—	—
Arkansas	169	103	151	312	327	358	415	441	420	365
California	230	186	156	166	287	237	243	234	195	161
Colorado	42	0	0	—	—	—	—	—	—	—
Connecticut	317	180	221	227	270	321	287	185	185	180
Delaware	20	18	17	17	19	30	32	30	30	28
District of Columbia	0	0	0	—	—	—	—	—	—	—
Florida	131	69	76	79	99	113	114	107	98	97
Georgia	138	102	87	94	88	—	0	—	—	—
Hawaii	0	0	0	—	—	—	—	—	—	—
Idaho	0	0	0	—	—	—	—	—	—	—
Illinois	1,136	714	345	260	358	369	301	297	327	252
Indiana	466	303	322	117	100	49	56	78	73	70
Iowa	364	206	261	167	207	302	334	386	410	287
Kansas	166	87	24	29	24	28	30	0	0	0
Kentucky	0	0	0	—	—	—	—	—	—	—
Louisiana	353	337	204	235	223	216	48	42	45	56
Maine	83	24	0	—	—	—	—	—	—	—
Maryland	315	99	118	134	157	128	167	206	204	183
Massachusetts	600	434	398	348	390	456	514	529	552	525
Michigan	364	304	244	154	154	196	295	313	255	245
Minnesota	97	0	0	—	—	—	—	—	—	—
Mississippi	0	0	0	—	—	—	—	—	—	—
Missouri	758	512	486	501	614	673	625	663	502	460
Montana	0	0	0	—	—	—	—	—	—	—
Nebraska	380	151	58	54	51	63	75	65	85	58
Nevada	0	0	0	—	—	—	—	—	—	—
New Hampshire	46	44	14	0	—	—	—	—	—	—
New Jersey	1,310	981	837	869	1,375	1,050	1,292	1,583	1,377	1,417
New Mexico	0	0	0	—	—	—	—	—	—	—
New York	938	655	470	422	510	460	482	417	315	233
North Carolina	268	167	114	178	255	354	290	284	282	353
North Dakota	122	59	0	—	—	—	—	—	—	—
Ohio	1,574	1,125	894	1,036	1,136	1,140	1,028	1,079	1,097	888
Oklahoma	0	0	0	—	—	—	—	—	—	—
Oregon	0	0	0	—	—	—	—	—	—	—
Pennsylvania	2,472	1,833	1,726	1,831	1,964	2,158	2,196	2,170	2,226	2,070
Rhode Island	76	69	41	37	31	32	45	40	41	48
South Carolina	6	13	9	—	—	—	—	—	—	—
South Dakota	84	32	104	56	23	—	—	—	—	—
Tennessee	753	451	302	416	511	487	437	488	578	792
Texas	144	110	130	139	200	192	208	240	231	232
Utah	0	0	0	—	—	—	—	—	—	—
Vermont	0	0	0	—	—	—	—	—	—	—
Virginia	407	289	298	319	415	476	499	522	427	407
Washington	0	0	0	—	—	—	—	—	—	—
West Virginia	109	61	151	80	82	85	80	87	86	78
Wisconsin	314	96	45	79	104	88	97	149	70	70
Wyoming	0	0	0	—	—	—	—	—	—	—
American Samoa	0	0	0	—	—	—	—	—	—	—
Guam	0	0	0	—	—	—	—	—	—	—
Puerto Rico	0	0	0	—	—	—	—	—	—	—
Virgin Islands	0	0	0	—	—	—	—	—	—	—

[1] National and regional totals exclude American Samoa, Guam, Puerto Rico, and the Virgin Islands.

Table 17
ENROLLMENTS IN BASIC RN PROGRAMS AND PERCENTAGE CHANGE FROM PREVIOUS YEAR, BY TYPE OF PROGRAM: 1975 TO 1994[1]

YEAR	ALL BASIC RN PROGRAMS		BACCALAUREATE PROGRAMS		ASSOCIATE DEGREE PROGRAMS		DIPLOMA PROGRAMS	
	Number of Enrollments	Percent Change	Number of Enrollments	Percent Change	Number of Enrollments	Percent Change	Number of Enrollments	Percent Change
1975	248,171	+2.3	99,837	+5.7	88,121	+4.7	60,213	-5.9
1976	247,044	-0.4	99,949	+0.1	91,004	+3.3	56,091	-6.8
1977	245,390	-0.7	101,430	+1.5	91,102	+0.1	52,858	-5.8
1978	239,486	-2.4	99,900	-1.5	91,527	+0.5	48,059	-9.1
1979	234,659	-2.0	98,939	-1.0	92,069	+0.6	43,651	-9.2
1980	230,966	-1.6	95,858	-3.1	94,060	+2.2	41,048	-6.0
1981	234,995	+1.7	93,967	-2.0	100,019	+6.3	41,009	-0.1
1982	242,035	+3.0	94,363	+0.4	105,324	+5.3	42,348	+3.3
1983	250,553	+3.5	98,941	+4.9	109,605	+4.1	42,007	-0.8
1984	237,232	-5.3	95,008	-4.0	104,968	-4.2	37,256	-11.3
1985	217,955	-8.1	91,020	-4.2	96,756	-7.8	30,179	-19.0
1986	193,712	-11.1	81,602	-10.3	89,469	-7.5	22,641	-25.0
1987	182,947	-5.6	73,621	-9.8	90,399	+1.0	18,927	-16.4
1988	184,924	+1.1	70,078	-4.8	95,986	+6.2	18,860	-0.4
1989	201,458	+8.9	74,865	+6.8	106,175	+10.6	20,418	+8.3
1990	221,170	+9.8	81,788	+9.2	117,413	+10.6	21,969	+7.6
1991	237,598	+7.4	90,877	+11.1	123,816	+5.4	22,905	+4.3
1992	257,983	+8.6	102,128	+12.4	132,603	+7.1	23,252	+1.5
1993	270,228	+4.7	110,693	+8.4	137,300	+3.5	22,235	-4.4
1994	268,350	-0.7	112,659	+1.8	135,895	-1.0	19,796	-11.0

[1] Excludes American Samoa, Guam, Puerto Rico, and the Virgin Islands.

Table 18
ENROLLMENTS IN PUBLIC AND PRIVATE BASIC RN PROGRAMS, BY TYPE OF PROGRAM: 1985 TO 1994[1]

PUBLIC AND PRIVATE NURSING PROGRAMS	TOTAL ENROLLMENTS									
	1985	1986	1987	1988	1989	1990	1991	1992	1993	1994
All Programs	217,955	193,715	182,947	184,924	201,458	221,170	237,598	257,983	270,228	268,350
Public	141,399	129,362	130,230	134,575	148,343	162,707	176,892	186,230	193,951	191,193
Private	76,556	64,350	52,717	50,349	53,115	58,463	60,706	71,753	76,277	77,157
Baccalaureate	91,020	81,602	73,621	70,078	74,865	81,788	90,877	102,128	110,693	112,659
Public	53,450	47,329	47,276	45,414	49,792	54,245	59,257	62,045	65,643	65,331
Private	37,570	34,273	26,345	24,664	25,073	27,543	31,620	40,083	45,050	47,328
Associate Degree	96,756	89,469	90,399	95,986	106,175	117,413	123,816	132,603	137,300	135,895
Public	83,693	78,207	79,542	85,413	94,501	104,311	112,576	120,030	123,794	122,061
Private	13,063	11,262	10,857	10,573	11,674	13,102	11,240	12,573	13,506	13,834
Diploma	30,179	22,641	18,927	18,860	20,418	21,969	22,905	23,252	22,235	19,796
Public	4,256	3,826	3,412	3,748	4,050	4,151	5,059	4,155	4,514	3,801
Private	25,923	18,815	15,515	15,112	16,368	17,818	17,846	19,097	17,721	15,995

[1] Excludes American Samoa, Guam, Puerto Rico, and the Virgin Islands.

Table 19
TOTAL ENROLLMENTS IN ALL BASIC RN PROGRAMS, BY NLN REGION AND STATE: 1985 TO 1994[1]

NLN REGION AND STATE	NUMBER OF TOTAL ENROLLMENTS									
	1985	1986	1987	1988	1989	1990	1991	1992	1993	1994
United States	**217,955**	**193,712**	**182,947**	**184,924**	**201,458**	**221,170**	**237,598**	**257,983**	**270,228**	**268,350**
North Atlantic	63,673	56,345	50,521	49,533	53,315	56,673	60,276	68,512	72,271	74,088
Midwest	63,247	54,591	50,450	49,957	53,665	59,682	64,100	67,540	71,221	71,004
South	63,911	58,316	57,674	60,912	68,882	77,851	84,704	92,796	97,530	94,284
West	27,124	24,460	24,302	24,522	25,596	26,964	28,518	29,135	29,206	28,974
Alabama	5,050	4,300	3,799	4,003	4,462	4,886	5,704	6,962	8,008	8,380
Alaska	377	455	268	269	274	268	231	228	224	269
Arizona	1,933	1,816	1,827	1,819	1,765	1,799	1,881	2,095	2,350	2,309
Arkansas	2,028	1,936	1,929	2,170	2,627	3,268	3,628	3,734	3,534	3,347
California	13,705	11,992	12,108	11,668	12,003	12,455	13,511	13,599	13,526	13,525
Colorado	1,546	1,446	1,393	1,336	1,592	1,706	1,823	1,937	2,096	1,903
Connecticut	2,995	2,551	2,267	2,268	2,371	2,506	2,784	2,734	2,760	2,796
Delaware	1,073	957	829	800	879	937	809	1,155	1,327	1,332
District of Columbia	1,251	1,055	754	799	704	710	759	877	983	1,051
Florida	6,398	5,545	5,475	5,877	6,371	7,181	7,800	8,166	8,510	8,918
Georgia	3,694	3,278	3,185	3,532	3,942	4,450	5,026	5,785	6,259	6,078
Hawaii	311	464	520	825	659	624	466	665	824	911
Idaho	467	470	550	625	710	885	722	684	692	704
Illinois	10,641	9,246	8,087	8,114	8,532	9,171	9,819	10,752	11,522	12,104
Indiana	6,280	6,260	5,830	6,007	6,219	7,916	8,027	6,871	7,093	7,370
Iowa	3,736	2,966	2,917	2,817	3,126	3,420	3,705	4,280	4,519	4,349
Kansas	2,255	1,775	1,791	1,951	2,272	2,721	2,725	3,015	3,125	3,072
Kentucky	3,724	3,521	3,550	3,801	4,250	4,515	5,527	5,914	5,663	5,594
Louisiana	4,779	5,081	4,957	5,462	7,163	7,620	7,604	10,336	12,240	10,130
Maine	1,017	910	1,001	984	1,153	1,350	1,508	1,827	1,969	1,934
Maryland	3,591	3,097	2,775	2,629	2,838	3,055	3,424	4,071	4,015	4,099
Massachusetts	8,190	7,119	6,239	5,593	6,232	6,513	7,062	7,883	8,313	8,334
Michigan	8,472	7,540	7,553	6,928	7,219	7,575	8,270	8,865	8,796	8,977
Minnesota	3,029	2,659	2,548	2,480	2,774	3,018	3,293	3,318	3,521	3,357
Mississippi	2,812	2,669	2,584	2,720	2,980	3,488	3,658	3,974	3,995	3,761
Missouri	4,799	4,218	3,875	3,702	3,943	4,421	5,032	5,956	6,337	6,017
Montana	947	887	739	868	896	916	888	994	974	915
Nebraska	2,413	1,266	1,169	1,196	1,603	2,011	2,369	2,535	2,552	2,458
Nevada	582	477	488	439	452	568	638	490	556	513
New Hampshire	1,076	819	803	805	905	1,116	1,243	1,408	1,422	1,418
New Jersey	6,792	5,942	5,410	5,642	5,959	6,418	7,140	7,788	7,886	7,698
New Mexico	971	757	920	987	1,072	1,220	1,337	1,386	1,347	1,428
New York	23,605	21,380	19,266	18,105	19,414	20,056	21,110	24,515	26,656	28,916
North Carolina	4,919	4,600	4,679	5,086	5,852	6,677	6,721	7,000	7,304	7,251
North Dakota	1,137	865	650	551	738	862	722	913	808	777
Ohio	12,722	11,156	10,651	10,748	11,464	11,866	12,523	13,450	14,218	14,487
Oklahoma	2,065	1,977	2,324	2,243	2,562	2,840	3,241	3,363	3,345	3,251
Oregon	2,075	1,676	1,620	1,595	1,747	1,851	2,012	1,967	1,480	1,680
Pennsylvania	15,759	13,832	12,325	13,106	14,159	15,294	15,776	18,069	18,596	18,009
Rhode Island	1,372	1,348	1,213	1,017	1,086	1,258	1,482	1,584	1,678	1,951
South Carolina	2,764	2,536	2,424	2,664	2,931	3,658	3,383	4,026	3,891	3,764
South Dakota	1,205	1,067	1,104	1,057	1,125	1,071	1,653	1,255	1,255	1,112
Tennessee	5,523	4,856	4,797	4,726	4,981	6,566	6,836	6,167	6,830	6,724
Texas	9,744	8,950	9,313	10,082	11,394	12,366	14,004	14,360	15,087	14,089
Utah	845	910	794	779	1,003	1,066	1,093	1,250	1,299	1,192
Vermont	543	432	414	414	453	515	603	672	681	649
Virginia	4,578	3,983	4,045	4,139	4,577	5,186	5,810	6,414	6,178	6,260
Washington	3,027	2,836	2,633	2,828	2,945	3,044	3,211	3,246	3,288	3,146
West Virginia	2,242	1,987	1,838	1,778	1,952	2,095	2,338	2,524	2,671	2,638
Wisconsin	6,558	5,573	4,275	4,406	4,650	5,630	5,962	6,330	7,475	6,924
Wyoming	338	337	442	484	478	562	705	594	550	479
American Samoa	11	14	16	16	16	16	13	16	11	11
Guam	60	60	60	—	19	20	69	69	68	113
Puerto Rico	3,144	3,642	3,561	2,918	2,980	3,408	3,120	3,575	4,157	3,754
Virgin Islands	55	56	73	50	47	55	55	75	77	111

[1] National and regional totals exclude American Samoa, Guam, Puerto Rico, and the Virgin Islands.

Table 20
TOTAL ENROLLMENTS IN BASIC BACCALAUREATE NURSING PROGRAMS, BY NLN REGION AND STATE: 1985 TO 1994[1]

NLN REGION AND STATE	NUMBER OF TOTAL ENROLLMENTS[2]									
	1985	1986	1987	1988	1989	1990	1991	1992	1993	1994
United States	**91,020**	**81,602**	**73,621**	**70,078**	**74,865**	**81,788**	**90,877**	**102,128**	**110,693**	**112,659**
North Atlantic	26,914	23,065	19,710	17,695	17,742	18,563	20,450	24,777	27,797	28,628
Midwest	27,013	24,620	21,823	21,183	21,916	24,164	27,762	29,691	32,253	33,649
South	25,849	23,998	22,564	22,134	25,846	28,978	31,823	36,418	39,622	38,817
West	11,244	9,919	9,524	9,066	9,361	10,083	10,842	11,242	11,021	11,565
Alabama	2,763	2,276	1,991	1,904	2,040	2,160	2,723	3,546	4,040	4,070
Alaska	317	329	203	203	199	182	151	156	156	212
Arizona	822	765	591	595	546	523	548	644	801	843
Arkansas	626	594	580	549	672	740	856	969	1,091	1,229
California	5,139	4,258	4,309	3,947	3,990	4,173	4,654	4,747	4,676	4,855
Colorado	781	725	711	585	756	871	963	1,111	1,108	981
Connecticut	1,481	1,281	1,076	1,012	988	1,136	1,114	1,260	1,420	1,463
Delaware	738	625	467	411	419	460	343	633	759	819
District of Columbia	1,045	843	675	647	552	564	669	801	886	955
Florida	1,757	1,540	1,430	1,418	1,494	1,567	1,809	2,020	1,873	2,328
Georgia	1,197	1,025	901	988	1,215	1,372	1,589	1,810	2,136	2,249
Hawaii	58	228	401	354	284	162	220	288	429	548
Idaho	37	32	107	183	223	369	189	187	209	215
Illinois	4,096	3,826	3,249	3,059	3,028	3,131	3,667	4,201	4,787	5,977
Indiana	3,100	3,586	3,351	3,418	3,321	4,155	4,711	3,344	3,441	3,614
Iowa	1,235	1,057	821	779	788	859	1,006	1,182	1,308	1,338
Kansas	1,106	863	780	836	940	1,137	1,230	1,520	1,549	1,613
Kentucky	1,482	1,652	1,477	1,571	1,846	1,721	2,191	2,304	1,934	2,013
Louisiana	3,086	3,397	3,361	3,623	5,127	5,595	5,214	7,465	8,530	7,280
Maine	566	523	700	666	797	912	1,018	1,157	1,313	1,305
Maryland	1,187	1,166	968	758	819	770	974	1,244	1,385	1,543
Massachusetts	3,999	3,394	2,970	2,578	2,821	2,770	3,030	3,599	3,887	4,000
Michigan	3,663	3,283	3,157	3,096	2,867	2,991	3,341	3,717	3,582	3,699
Minnesota	1,275	1,138	1,046	844	895	903	1,072	1,140	1,307	1,159
Mississippi	1,005	1,179	998	958	995	1,311	1,428	1,494	1,399	1,170
Missouri	1,499	1,366	1,217	1,057	1,035	1,329	1,778	2,610	2,850	2,527
Montana	740	659	565	606	621	672	648	749	741	622
Nebraska	1,160	748	824	1,026	1,295	1,514	1,808	1,914	1,929	1,872
Nevada	236	181	193	231	281	338	376	255	267	271
New Hampshire	515	432	363	329	352	389	482	523	567	582
New Jersey	1,997	1,792	1,480	1,056	1,251	1,313	1,424	1,590	1,662	1,672
New Mexico	284	211	190	181	174	208	318	377	329	352
New York	8,313	6,826	5,793	4,981	4,603	4,389	5,000	6,469	7,701	8,158
North Carolina	1,831	1,623	1,563	1,348	1,409	1,776	1,745	2,081	2,265	2,239
North Dakota	693	606	537	551	738	862	722	913	808	777
Ohio	4,408	3,997	3,781	3,571	3,789	3,950	4,210	5,137	5,696	6,313
Oklahoma	877	740	933	780	947	1,076	1,271	1,357	1,266	1,233
Oregon	890	744	665	616	666	745	905	922	412	773
Pennsylvania	7,219	6,344	5,288	5,364	5,330	5,812	6,327	7,528	8,286	8,405
Rhode Island	750	754	682	470	461	616	809	966	1,060	1,019
South Carolina	1,411	1,195	994	997	1,049	1,139	1,337	1,777	1,753	1,774
South Dakota	688	624	594	555	632	606	1,165	744	592	554
Tennessee	1,980	1,785	1,667	1,629	1,662	2,547	2,418	1,868	2,544	2,761
Texas	4,262	3,792	3,747	3,676	4,238	4,492	5,350	5,224	5,890	5,371
Utah	450	407	395	378	415	523	442	515	544	576
Vermont	291	251	216	181	168	202	234	251	256	250
Virginia	1,736	1,488	1,339	1,327	1,611	1,850	1,911	2,165	2,255	2,255
Washington	1,312	1,179	977	962	971	1,079	1,179	1,166	1,227	1,194
West Virginia	649	546	615	608	722	862	1,007	1,094	1,261	1,302
Wisconsin	4,090	3,526	2,466	2,391	2,588	2,727	3,052	3,269	4,404	4,206
Wyoming	178	201	217	225	235	238	249	125	122	123
American Samoa	0	0	0	—	—	—	—	—	—	—
Guam	0	0	0	—	19	20	69	69	68	113
Puerto Rico	2,292	2,708	2,615	2,118	1,873	1,952	1,672	1,937	2,213	2,236
Virgin Islands	28	26	46	27	26	38	41	54	41	80

[1]National and regional totals exclude American Samoa, Guam, Puerto Rico, and the Virgin Islands.
[2]Includes basic students only.

Table 21
TOTAL ENROLLMENTS IN ASSOCIATE DEGREE NURSING PROGRAMS, BY NLN REGION AND STATE: 1985 TO 1994[1]

NLN REGION AND STATE	NUMBER OF TOTAL ENROLLMENTS									
	1985	1986	1987	1988	1989	1990	1991	1992	1993	1994
United States	**96,756**	**89,469**	**90,399**	**95,986**	**106,175**	**117,413**	**123,816**	**132,603**	**137,300**	**135,895**
North Atlantic	24,468	23,213	22,296	23,044	25,932	27,695	28,983	32,747	34,038	35,660
Midwest	24,326	22,013	22,497	23,215	26,084	29,737	30,330	31,590	32,876	32,385
South	32,637	30,104	31,166	34,576	38,281	43,550	47,296	50,835	52,583	50,773
West	15,325	14,139	14,440	15,151	15,878	16,431	17,207	17,431	17,803	17,077
Alabama	2,065	1,900	1,742	2,039	2,363	2,648	2,881	3,319	3,885	4,281
Alaska	60	63	65	66	75	86	80	72	68	57
Arizona	1,111	1,051	1,236	1,224	1,219	1,276	1,333	1,451	1,549	1,466
Arkansas	1,067	1,012	927	997	1,225	1,486	1,591	1,542	1,499	1,381
California	8,091	7,344	7,461	7,416	7,656	7,832	8,388	8,390	8,468	8,338
Colorado	685	709	682	751	836	835	860	826	988	922
Connecticut	875	742	680	703	761	638	1,038	1,113	970	976
Delaware	285	285	320	343	417	427	408	449	493	440
District of Columbia	206	212	79	152	152	146	90	76	97	96
Florida	4,423	3,854	3,905	4,299	4,672	5,383	5,799	5,966	6,446	6,399
Georgia	2,124	1,971	2,045	2,323	2,584	3,010	3,419	3,975	4,123	3,829
Hawaii	253	236	119	471	375	462	246	377	395	363
Idaho	430	438	443	442	487	516	533	497	483	489
Illinois	4,677	4,243	4,020	4,349	4,835	5,359	5,524	5,806	5,955	5,479
Indiana	2,217	1,954	1,969	2,339	2,695	3,604	3,125	3,297	3,363	3,493
Iowa	1,664	1,360	1,685	1,603	1,808	1,910	1,929	2,161	2,323	2,294
Kansas	994	822	947	1,063	1,269	1,512	1,446	1,465	1,576	1,459
Kentucky	2,242	1,869	2,073	2,230	2,404	2,794	3,336	3,610	3,729	3,581
Louisiana	1937	973	993	1,260	1,510	1,676	2,168	2,797	3,633	2,769
Maine	326	329	284	318	356	438	490	670	656	629
Maryland	1,988	1,669	1,574	1,608	1,714	1,953	2,104	2,473	2,272	2,246
Massachusetts	2,689	2,586	2,328	2,274	2,560	2,718	2,876	3,068	3,202	3,148
Michigan	4,179	3,753	4,020	3,495	4,009	4,217	4,504	4,679	4,729	4,866
Minnesota	1,549	1,457	1,502	1,636	1,879	2,115	2,221	2,178	2,214	2,198
Mississippi	1,774	1,490	1,586	1,762	1,985	2,177	2,230	2,480	2,596	2,591
Missouri	1,727	1,617	1,567	1,561	1,664	1,857	2,032	2,260	2,479	2,689
Montana	207	228	174	262	275	244	240	245	233	293
Nebraska	357	112	156	97	232	414	478	520	498	483
Nevada	346	296	295	208	171	230	262	235	289	242
New Hampshire	456	328	401	467	553	727	761	885	855	836
New Jersey	2,418	2,069	2,048	2,280	2,311	2,455	2,707	2,932	2,946	2,909
New Mexico	687	546	730	806	898	1,012	1,019	1,009	1,018	1,076
New York	13,324	13,021	12,339	12,151	13,710	14,555	15,132	17,154	18,417	20,263
North Carolina	2,812	2,648	2,789	3,362	3,877	4,238	4,313	4,262	4,311	4,337
North Dakota	167	126	85	—	—	—	—	—	—	—
Ohio	4,606	4,453	4,478	4,826	5,332	5,580	5,900	5,933	6,311	6,283
Oklahoma	1,188	1,237	1,391	1,463	1,615	1,764	1,970	2,006	2,079	2,018
Oregon	1,185	932	955	979	1,081	1,106	1,107	1,045	1,068	907
Pennsylvania	3,207	3,007	3,202	3,659	4,280	4,722	4,536	5,463	5,468	5,146
Rhode Island	430	453	417	464	547	556	576	516	509	818
South Carolina	1,321	1,313	1,421	1,667	1,882	2,519	2,046	2,249	2,138	1,990
South Dakota	356	348	414	383	445	444	488	511	663	558
Tennessee	2,167	2,170	2,302	2,381	2,476	3,046	3,292	3,118	3,102	2,920
Texas	5,245	4,951	5,340	6,142	6,830	7,482	8,225	8,698	8,760	8,297
Utah	395	503	399	401	588	543	651	735	755	616
Vermont	252	181	198	233	285	313	369	421	425	399
Virginia	1,976	1,813	2,015	2,038	2,075	2,299	2,743	3,061	2,755	2,935
Washington	1,715	1,657	1,656	1,866	1974	1,965	2,032	2,080	2,061	1,952
West Virginia	1,308	1,234	1,063	1,005	1,069	1,075	1,179	1,279	1,255	1,199
Wisconsin	1,833	1,768	1,654	1,863	1,916	2,725	2,683	2,780	2,765	2,583
Wyoming	160	136	225	259	243	324	456	469	428	356
American Samoa	11	14	16	16	16	16	13	16	11	11
Guam	60	60	60	—	—	—	—	—	—	—
Puerto Rico	852	934	946	800	1,107	1,456	1,448	1,638	1,944	1,518
Virgin Islands	27	30	27	23	21	17	14	21	36	31

[1] National and regional totals exclude American Samoa, Guam, Puerto Rico, and the Virgin Islands.

Table 22
TOTAL ENROLLMENTS IN DIPLOMA NURSING PROGRAMS, BY NLN REGION AND STATE: 1985 TO 1994[1]

NLN REGION AND STATE	NUMBER OF TOTAL ENROLLMENTS									
	1985	1986	1987	1988	1989	1990	1991	1992	1993	1994
United States	**30,179**	**22,641**	**18,927**	**18,860**	**20,418**	**21,969**	**22,905**	**23,252**	**22,235**	**19,796**
North Atlantic	12,291	10,067	8,515	8,794	9,641	10,415	10,843	10,988	10,436	9,800
Midwest	11,908	7,958	6,130	5,559	5,665	5,781	6,008	6,259	6,092	4,970
South	5,425	4,214	3,944	4,202	4,755	5,323	5,585	5,543	5,325	4,694
West	555	402	338	305	357	450	469	462	382	332
Alabama	222	124	66	60	59	78	100	97	83	29
Alaska	0	0	0	—	—	—	—	—	—	—
Arizona	0	0	0	—	—	—	—	—	—	—
Arkansas	335	330	422	624	730	1,042	1,181	1,223	944	737
California	475	390	338	305	357	450	469	462	382	332
Colorado	80	12	0	—	—	—	—	—	—	—
Connecticut	639	528	511	553	622	732	632	361	370	357
Delaware	50	47	42	46	43	50	58	73	75	73
District of Columbia	0	0	0	—	—	—	—	—	—	—
Florida	218	151	140	160	205	231	192	180	191	191
Georgia	373	282	239	221	143	68	18	—	—	—
Hawaii	0	0	0	—	—	—	—	—	—	—
Idaho	0	0	0	—	—	—	—	—	—	—
Illinois	1,868	1,177	818	706	669	681	628	745	780	648
Indiana	963	720	510	250	203	157	191	230	289	263
Iowa	837	549	411	435	530	651	770	937	888	717
Kansas	155	90	64	52	63	72	49	30	—	—
Kentucky	0	0	0	—	—	—	—	—	—	—
Louisiana	756	711	603	579	526	349	222	74	77	81
Maine	125	58	17	—	—	—	—	—	—	—
Maryland	416	262	233	263	305	332	346	354	358	310
Massachusetts	1,502	1,139	941	741	851	1,025	1,156	1,216	1,224	1,186
Michigan	630	504	376	337	343	367	425	469	485	412
Minnesota	205	64	0	—	—	—	—	—	—	—
Mississippi	33	0	0	—	—	—	—	—	—	—
Missouri	1,573	1,235	1,091	1,084	1,244	1,235	1,222	1,086	1,008	801
Montana	0	0	0	—	—	—	—	—	—	—
Nebraska	896	406	189	73	76	83	83	101	125	103
Nevada	0	0	0	—	—	—	—	—	—	—
New Hampshire	105	59	39	9	—	—	—	—	—	—
New Jersey	2,377	2,081	1,882	2,306	2,397	2,650	3,009	3,266	3,278	3,117
New Mexico	0	0	0	—	—	—	—	—	—	—
New York	1,968	1,533	1,134	973	1,101	1,112	978	892	538	495
North Carolina	276	329	327	376	566	663	663	657	728	675
North Dakota	277	133	28	—	—	—	—	—	—	—
Ohio	3,708	2,706	2,392	2,351	2,343	2,336	2,413	2,380	2,211	1,891
Oklahoma	0	0	0	—	—	—	—	—	—	—
Oregon	0	0	0	—	—	—	—	—	—	—
Pennsylvania	5,333	4,481	3,835	4,083	4,549	4,760	4,913	5,078	4,842	4,458
Rhode Island	192	141	114	83	78	86	97	102	109	114
South Carolina	32	28	9	—	—	—	—	—	—	—
South Dakota	161	95	96	119	48	21	—	—	—	—
Tennessee	1,376	901	828	716	843	973	1,126	1,181	1,184	1,043
Texas	237	207	226	264	326	392	429	438	437	421
Utah	0	0	0	—	—	—	—	—	—	—
Vermont	0	0	0	—	—	—	—	—	—	—
Virginia	866	682	691	774	891	1,037	1,156	1,188	1,168	1,070
Washington	0	0	0	—	—	—	—	—	—	—
West Virginia	285	207	160	165	161	158	152	151	155	137
Wisconsin	635	279	155	152	146	178	227	281	306	135
Wyoming	0	0	0	—	—	—	—	—	—	—
American Samoa	0	0	0	—	—	—	0	—	—	—
Guam	0	0	0	—	—	—	0	—	—	—
Puerto Rico	0	0	0	—	—	—	0	—	—	—
Virgin Islands	0	0	0	—	—	—	0	—	—	—

[1] National and regional totals exclude American Samoa, Guam, Puerto Rico, and the Virgin Islands.

Table 23
BASIC AND RN STUDENT ENROLLMENTS IN BACCALAUREATE NURSING PROGRAMS: 1985 TO 1994[1]

YEAR	ENROLLMENTS IN BACCALAUREATE NURSING PROGRAMS			
	Total Enrollments	Basic Programs		BRN* Programs
		Basic Students	RN Students	RN Students
1985	133,960	91,020	22,812	20,128
1986	127,957	81,602	25,247	21,108
1987	119,996	73,621	26,503	19,872
1988	113,105	70,078	25,597	17,430
1989	116,539	74,865	24,524	17,150
1990	122,504	81,788	23,777	16,939
1991	130,195	90,877	22,634	16,684
1992	142,494	102,128	22,399	17,967
1993	151,566	110,693	23,075	17,798
1994	155,655	112,659	25,536	17,460

[1] Excludes American Samoa, Guam, Puerto Rico, and the Virgin Islands.
* BRN programs are baccalaureate programs that admit only RNs.

Table 24
FULL-TIME AND PART-TIME ENROLLMENTS OF BASIC AND RN STUDENTS IN BACCALAUREATE NURSING PROGRAMS: 1990 TO 1994[1]

YEAR AND TYPE OF STUDENT	ENROLLMENTS IN BACCALAUREATE NURSING PROGRAMS		
	Total	Full Time	Part Time
1990 (Total)	**122,504**	**78,985**	**43,519**
Basic Students	81,788	69,799	11,989
RNs in Basic Programs	23,777	4,160	19,617
RNs in BRN* Programs	16,939	5,026	11,913
1991 (Total)	**130,195**	**86,094**	**44,101**
Basic Students	90,877	77,152	13,725
RNs in Basic Programs	22,634	6,016	16,618
RNs in BRN* Programs	16,684	2,926	13,758
1992 (Total)	**142,494**	**95,745**	**46,749**
Basic Students	102,128	88,002	14,126
RNs in Basic Programs	22,399	4,353	18,046
RNs in BRN* Programs	17,967	3,390	14,577
1993 (Total)	**151,566**	**104,793**	**46,773**
Basic Students	110,693	96,316	14,377
RNs in Basic Programs	23,075	4,617	18,458
RNs in BRN* Programs	17,798	3,860	13,938
1994 (Total)	**155,655**	**105,021**	**50,634**
Basic Students	112,659	96,653	16,006
RNs in Basic Programs	25,536	4,549	20,987
RNs in BRN* Programs	17,460	3,819	13,641

[1] Excludes American Samoa, Guam, Puerto Rico, and the Virgin Islands.
*BRN programs are baccalaureate programs that admit only RNs.

Table 25
TOTAL ENROLLMENTS IN BACCALAUREATE NURSING PROGRAMS, BY NLN REGION AND STATE: 1990 TO 1994[1]

NLN REGION AND STATE	ENROLLMENTS IN BACCALAUREATE NURSING PROGRAMS [2]									
	1990		1991		1992		1993		1994	
	Total	RNs Only	Total	RNs Only	Total	RNs Only	Total	RNs Only	Total	RNs Only
United States	**122,504**	**40,716**	**130,195**	**39,318**	**142,494**	**40,366**	**151,566**	**40,873**	**155,655**	**42,996**
North Atlantic	33,057	14,494	34,768	14,318	39,973	15,196	43,267	15,470	46,490	17,862
Midwest	35,933	11,769	38,916	11,154	40,577	10,886	43,225	10,972	45,071	11,422
South	36,963	7,985	39,761	7,938	44,153	7,735	47,651	8,029	47,656	8,839
West	16,551	6,468	16,750	5,908	17,791	6,549	17,423	6,402	16,438	4,873
Alabama	2,614	454	3,173	450	3,969	423	4,424	384	4,501	431
Alaska	218	36	165	14	167	11	165	9	222	10
Arizona	1,243	720	1,493	945	1,767	1,123	2,062	1,261	2,350	1,507
Arkansas	799	59	930	74	1,072	103	1,188	97	1,366	137
California	8,101	3,928	8,015	3,361	8,197	3,450	7,988	3,312	5,990	1,135
Colorado	1,405	534	1,314	351	1,602	491	1,642	534	1,594	613
Connecticut	1,704	568	1,851	737	1,963	703	2,182	762	2,415	952
Delaware	699	239	618	275	996	363	1,289	530	1,545	726
District of Columbia	680	116	769	100	916	115	968	82	1,032	77
Florida	2,806	1,239	3,114	1,305	3,247	1,227	3,229	1,356	3,868	1,540
Georgia	1,865	493	2,055	466	2,313	503	2,702	566	2,879	630
Hawaii	345	183	398	178	422	134	562	133	673	125
Idaho	530	161	272	83	310	123	339	130	339	124
Illinois	4,642	1,511	5,030	1,363	5,703	1,502	6,176	1,389	7,466	1,489
Indiana	5,250	1,095	5,748	1,037	4,360	1,016	4,427	986	4,694	1,080
Iowa	1,496	637	1,624	618	2,043	861	2,311	1,003	1,876	538
Kansas	1,658	521	1,733	503	2,151	631	2,148	599	2,234	621
Kentucky	2,490	769	2,872	681	2,825	521	2,494	560	2,456	443
Louisiana	5,890	295	5,531	317	7,803	338	8,867	337	7,694	414
Maine	1,132	220	1,241	223	1,575	418	1,825	512	1,872	567
Maryland	1,367	597	1,527	553	1,939	695	1,995	610	2,170	627
Massachusetts	4,319	1,549	4,808	1,778	5,261	1,662	5,177	1,290	5,820	1,820
Michigan	4,873	1,882	5,206	1,865	5,354	1,637	5,187	1,605	5,101	1,402
Minnesota	1,512	609	1,701	629	1,706	566	1,875	568	1,775	616
Mississippi	1,447	136	1,511	83	1,573	79	1,515	116	1,368	198
Missouri	2,509	1,180	3,141	1,363	3,941	1,331	4,148	1,298	4,470	1,943
Montana	705	33	686	38	783	34	770	29	727	105
Nebraska	2,216	702	2,415	607	2,376	462	2,430	501	2,256	384
Nevada	454	116	440	64	302	47	311	44	308	37
New Hampshire	569	180	756	274	744	221	826	259	1,212	630
New Jersey	2,649	1,336	2,772	1,348	2,932	1,342	3,020	1,358	3,301	1,629
New Mexico	413	205	571	253	639	262	593	264	626	274
New York	110,818	6,429	10,979	5,979	12,938	6,469	14,378	6,677	14,916	6,758
North Carolina	2,285	509	2,362	617	2,793	712	3,005	740	3,059	820
North Dakota	956	94	822	100	974	61	859	51	877	100
Ohio	6,177	2,227	6,114	1,904	7,011	1,874	7,486	1,790	8,376	2,063
Oklahoma	1,287	211	1,455	184	1,501	144	1,403	137	1,393	160
Oregon	834	89	986	81	1,123	201	431	19	958	185
Pennsylvania	9,400	3,588	9,610	3,283	11,089	3,561	11,968	3,682	12,808	4,403
Rhode Island	770	154	956	147	1,122	156	1,169	109	1,152	133
South Carolina	1,441	302	1,640	303	2,026	249	2,053	300	2,064	290
South Dakota	756	150	1,418	253	872	128	825	233	673	119
Tennessee	3,267	720	3,122	704	2,472	604	3,171	627	3,481	720
Texas	5,631	1,139	6,287	937	6,156	932	6,939	1,049	6,365	994
Utah	661	138	612	170	732	217	803	259	833	257
Vermont	317	115	408	174	437	186	465	209	417	167
Virginia	2,483	633	2,735	824	2,896	731	2,993	738	3,212	957
Washington	1,376	297	1,524	345	1,615	449	1,627	400	1,683	489
West Virginia	1,291	429	1,447	440	1,568	474	1,673	412	1,780	478
Wisconsin	3,888	1,161	3,964	912	4,086	817	5,353	949	5,273	1,067
Wyoming	266	28	274	25	132	7	130	8	135	12
American Samoa	—	—	—	—	—	—	—	—	—	—
Guam	36	16	108	39	69	0	79	11	123	10
Puerto Rico	2,277	325	1,966	294	2,253	316	2,471	258	2,517	281
Virgin Islands	43	5	52	11	60	6	45	4	91	11

[1] National and regional totals exclude American Samoa, Guam, Puerto Rico, and the Virgin Islands.
[2] Totals include RNs in basic programs, RNs in BRN programs, and basic BSN students.

Table 26
GRADUATIONS FROM BASIC RN PROGRAMS AND PERCENTAGE CHANGE FROM PREVIOUS YEAR, BY TYPE OF PROGRAM: 1974-75 TO 1993-94[1]

ACADEMIC YEAR	ALL BASIC RN PROGRAMS		BACCALAUREATE PROGRAMS		ASSOCIATE DEGREE PROGRAMS		DIPLOMA PROGRAMS	
	Number of Graduations	Percent Change	Number of Graduations	Percent Change	Number of Graduations	Percent Change	Number of Graduations	Percent Change
1974-75	73,915	+10.2	20,170	+18.9	32,183	+11.3	21,562	+1.8
1975-76	77,065	+4.3	22,579	+11.9	34,625	+7.6	19,861	-7.9
1976-77	77,755	+0.9	23,452	+3.9	36,289	+4.8	18,014	-9.3
1977-78	77,874	+0.1	24,187	+3.1	36,556	+0.7	17,131	-4.9
1978-79	77,132	-1.0	25,048	+3.6	36,264	-0.8	15,820	-7.7
1979-80	75,523	-2.1	24,994	-0.2	36,034	-0.6	14,495	-8.4
1980-81	73,985	-2.0	24,370	-2.5	36,712	+1.9	12,903	-11.0
1981-82	74,052	+0.1	24,081	-1.2	38,289	+4.3	11,682	-9.5
1982-83	77,408	+4.5	23,855	-0.9	41,849	+9.3	11,704	+0.2
1983-84	80,312	+3.8	23,718	-0.6	44,394	+6.1	12,200	+4.2
1984-85	82,075	+2.2	24,975	+5.3	45,208	+1.8	11,892	-2.5
1985-86	77,027	-6.2	25,170	+0.8	41,333	-8.6	10,524	-11.5
1986-87	70,561	-8.4	23,761	-5.6	38,528	-6.8	8,272	-21.4
1987-88	64,839	-8.0	21,504	-9.5	37,397	-2.9	5,938	-28.2
1988-89	61,660	-4.9	18,997	-11.6	37,837	+1.2	4,826	-18.7
1989-90	66,088	+7.2	18,571	-2.2	42,318	+11.8	5,199	+7.7
1990-91	72,230	+9.3	19,264	+3.7	46,794	+10.6	6,172	+18.7
1991-92	80,839	+11.9	21,415	+11.2	52,896	+13.0	6,528	+5.8
1992-93	88,149	+9.0	24,442	+14.1	56,770	+7.3	6,937	+6.3
1993-94	94,870	+7.6	28,912	+18.3	58,839	+3.6	7,119	+2.6

[1] Excludes American Samoa, Guam, Puerto Rico, and the Virgin Islands.

Table 27
GRADUATIONS FROM PUBLIC AND PRIVATE BASIC RN PROGRAMS, BY TYPE OF PROGRAM: 1984-85 TO 1993-94[1]

PUBLIC AND PRIVATE NURSING PROGRAMS	NUMBER OF GRADUATIONS									
	1984-85	1985-86	1986-87	1987-88	1988-89	1989-90	1990-91	1991-92	1992-93	1993-94
All Programs	**82,075**	**77,027**	**70,561**	**64,839**	**61,660**	**66,088**	**72,230**	**80,839**	**88,149**	**94,870**
Public	56,216	54,456	50,865	48,608	47,644	51,926	57,892	64,405	70,152	73,610
Private	25,859	22,571	19,696	16,231	14,016	14,162	14,338	16,434	17,997	21,260
Baccalaureate	24,975	25,170	23,761	21,504	18,997	18,571	19,264	21,415	24,442	28,912
Public	15,176	15,977	14,746	13,568	12,203	12,434	13,073	14,498	16,588	18,902
Private	9,799	9,193	9,015	7,936	6,794	6,137	6,191	6,917	7,854	10,010
Associate Degree	45,208	41,333	38,528	37,397	37,837	42,318	46,794	52,896	56,770	58,839
Public	39,521	36,806	34,696	33,795	34,460	38,439	43,337	48,535	52,017	53,294
Private	5,687	4,527	3,832	3,602	3,377	3,879	3,457	4,361	4,753	5,545
Diploma	11,892	10,524	8,272	5,938	4,826	5,199	6,172	6,528	6,937	7,119
Public	1,519	1,673	1,423	1,245	981	1,053	1,482	1,372	1,547	1,414
Private	10,373	8,851	6,849	4,693	3,845	4,146	4,690	5,156	5,390	5,705

[1] Excludes American Samoa, Guam, Puerto Rico, and the Virgin Islands.

Table 28
GRADUATIONS FROM ALL BASIC RN PROGRAMS, BY NLN REGION AND STATE: 1984-85 TO 1993-94[1]

NLN REGION AND STATE	NUMBER OF GRADUATIONS									
	1984-85	1985-86	1986-87	1987-88	1988-89	1989-90	1990-91	1991-92	1992-93	1993-94
United States	**82,075**	**77,027**	**70,561**	**64,839**	**61,660**	**66,088**	**72,230**	**80,839**	**88,149**	**94,870**
North Atlantic	20,484	19,622	18,274	16,617	15,054	15,347	16,278	18,762	20,116	21,414
Midwest	25,208	23,378	20,664	18,072	17,264	18,354	19,961	21,900	24,137	25,713
South	25,181	23,250	21,397	20,123	19,768	21,982	25,214	28,622	32,047	35,133
West	11,202	10,777	10,226	10,027	9,574	10,405	10,777	11,555	11,849	12,610
Alabama	2,094	1,857	1,587	1,430	1,354	1,425	1,565	1,867	1,970	2,642
Alaska	78	61	51	46	64	62	51	77	78	79
Arizona	878	797	795	767	784	807	796	792	918	1,064
Arkansas	778	771	726	685	687	878	1,039	1,224	1,216	1,254
California	5,679	5,566	5,125	4,969	4,716	4,956	5,045	5,245	5,295	5,591
Colorado	667	585	521	552	524	584	751	845	912	966
Connecticut	1,003	917	814	733	663	710	737	878	811	823
Delaware	334	311	308	278	267	273	272	284	277	358
District of Columbia	352	332	279	246	231	191	169	188	181	234
Florida	3,272	2,995	2,655	2,715	2,504	2,677	3,064	3,496	3,834	4,025
Georgia	1,731	1,547	1,432	1,236	1,206	1,446	1,604	1,848	2,164	2,467
Hawaii	129	172	133	202	170	250	296	240	276	259
Idaho	257	249	212	228	214	270	291	336	318	325
Illinois	4,299	4,012	3,370	2,974	2,822	2,945	3,164	3,266	4,131	4,152
Indiana	2,131	2,230	2,026	1,755	1,734	1,747	1,881	2,034	2,236	2,537
Iowa	1,776	1,566	1,385	1,135	1,173	1,234	1,293	1,483	1,585	1,656
Kansas	1,229	1,051	915	843	812	1,171	1,214	1,191	1,312	1,359
Kentucky	1,325	1,287	1,092	1,148	1,193	1,253	1,424	1,674	1,994	2,190
Louisiana	939	1,000	998	999	994	980	1,216	1,201	1,700	1,811
Maine	372	379	364	288	310	269	326	400	483	594
Maryland	1,490	1,357	1,205	1,026	920	1,013	1,107	1,323	1,463	1,665
Massachusetts	2,736	2,420	2,386	2,029	1,685	1,726	1,865	2,016	2,272	2,536
Michigan	3,552	3,136	3,119	2,763	2,701	2,583	2,688	3,016	3,259	3,322
Minnesota	1,730	1,500	1,246	1,125	1,141	1,170	1,385	1,502	1,599	1,664
Mississippi	1,033	1,013	1,035	851	799	911	1,147	1,226	1,369	1,571
Missouri	1,947	1,859	1,461	1,397	1,358	1,456	1,771	1,963	2,175	2,479
Montana	244	258	245	203	208	225	207	243	215	267
Nebraska	819	503	430	288	321	347	430	613	703	844
Nevada	186	171	153	182	149	153	173	236	228	266
New Hampshire	383	334	311	305	275	313	331	359	503	485
New Jersey	2,010	2,072	1,863	1,678	1,570	1,640	1,766	2,027	2,258	2,372
New Mexico	363	407	430	385	418	550	499	534	566	601
New York	7,114	6,812	6,467	6,052	5,712	5,582	5,905	6,867	7,116	7,402
North Carolina	2,598	1,967	1,759	1,722	1,760	2,005	2,342	2,547	2,910	3,063
North Dakota	416	419	310	179	202	186	215	271	288	294
Ohio	4,748	4,782	4,355	3,753	3,459	3,726	3,898	4,350	4,566	4,874
Oklahoma	840	782	805	786	902	881	1,088	1,181	1,282	1,413
Oregon	757	740	748	755	643	697	670	776	838	782
Pennsylvania	5,441	5,304	4,844	4,459	3,835	4,139	4,315	5,141	5,568	5,763
Rhode Island	521	532	457	404	393	364	439	430	421	625
South Carolina	901	889	884	846	863	886	1,056	1,096	1,217	1,257
South Dakota	434	421	324	378	322	365	442	441	414	463
Tennessee	1,912	1,850	1,673	1,431	1,296	1,436	1,571	1,936	2,252	2,411
Texas	3,652	3,425	3,347	3,186	3,320	3,951	4,605	5,314	5,720	6,049
Utah	542	373	402	454	477	475	600	664	644	730
Vermont	218	209	181	145	113	140	153	172	226	222
Virginia	1,745	1,677	1,465	1,459	1,356	1,516	1,618	1,913	2,082	2,374
Washington	1,291	1,263	1,293	1,149	1,056	1,185	1,195	1,309	1,287	1,429
West Virginia	871	833	734	603	614	724	768	776	874	941
Wisconsin	2,127	1,899	1,723	1,482	1,219	1,424	1,580	1,770	1,869	2,069
Wyoming	131	135	118	135	151	191	203	258	274	251
American Samoa	11	10	10	10	10	12	13	12	6	6
Guam	12	12	12	—	0	20	0	0	7	16
Puerto Rico	1,286	1,017	1,045	908	962	1,022	989	914	951	915
Virgin Islands	12	13	12	17	11	6	12	14	10	14

[1] National and regional totals exclude American Samoa, Guam, Puerto Rico, and the Virgin Islands.

Table 29
GRADUATIONS FROM BASIC BACCALAUREATE NURSING PROGRAMS, BY NLN REGION AND STATE: 1984-85 TO 1993-94[1]

NLN REGION AND STATE	NUMBER OF GRADUATIONS[2]									
	1984-85	1985-86	1986-87	1987-88	1988-89	1989-90	1990-91	1991-92	1992-93	1993-94
United States	**24,975**	**25,170**	**23,761**	**21,504**	**18,997**	**18,571**	**19,264**	**21,415**	**24,442**	**28,912**
North Atlantic	6,915	6,744	6,320	5,720	4,802	4,208	4,001	4,294	4,959	5,793
Midwest	7,479	7,600	7,218	6,430	5,756	5,670	5,861	6,523	7,364	8,856
South	7,535	7,562	6,970	6,423	5,804	5,868	6,521	7,570	8,794	10,433
West	3,046	3,264	3,253	2,931	2,635	2,825	2,881	3,028	3,325	3,830
Alabama	955	781	688	568	511	491	481	522	553	912
Alaska	38	38	26	26	34	32	21	32	48	46
Arizona	310	251	279	247	230	240	201	186	241	269
Arkansas	185	207	188	200	152	196	185	241	256	297
California	1,252	1,362	1,394	1,283	1,163	1,242	1,221	1,184	1,285	1,500
Colorado	250	266	179	210	179	235	297	364	414	461
Connecticut	359	363	302	286	260	233	214	287	278	292
Delaware	180	166	167	137	105	93	67	90	85	121
District of Columbia	293	294	218	191	176	146	125	170	155	200
Florida	630	570	561	521	503	513	500	619	724	695
Georgia	467	425	446	415	326	397	453	483	582	777
Hawaii	0	65	89	90	40	72	134	66	96	98
Idaho	33	31	34	26	32	56	71	80	74	73
Illinois	1,171	1,185	1,156	984	943	929	841	892	1,019	1,345
Indiana	739	899	784	774	701	641	632	722	796	975
Iowa	432	438	410	322	254	231	239	271	304	324
Kansas	491	447	408	291	281	345	386	395	536	590
Kentucky	229	498	319	365	342	331	308	359	464	553
Louisiana	401	438	450	490	505	472	608	601	818	872
Maine	144	171	176	166	159	107	140	165	198	252
Maryland	404	393	379	345	282	262	278	356	390	532
Massachusetts	1,032	917	862	796	631	598	531	591	684	811
Michigan	898	902	897	850	862	728	753	801	969	933
Minnesota	582	507	466	415	322	339	389	427	540	578
Mississippi	337	356	359	309	208	250	322	395	425	507
Missouri	458	432	319	352	333	323	333	459	575	710
Montana	166	175	174	144	139	137	100	140	109	152
Nebraska	264	160	152	185	192	227	259	367	391	548
Nevada	38	43	33	35	34	45	61	89	99	98
New Hampshire	142	124	118	97	86	76	81	77	119	120
New Jersey	387	419	413	382	347	318	294	265	339	391
New Mexico	67	86	73	71	50	58	46	59	69	93
New York	2,166	1,982	1,959	1,724	1,468	1,227	1,092	1,131	1,305	1,628
North Carolina	663	626	558	508	440	369	450	586	702	724
North Dakota	163	192	198	179	202	186	215	271	288	294
Ohio	1,209	1,315	1,326	1,198	1,006	1,008	1,003	1,012	1,116	1,477
Oklahoma	306	339	314	254	327	270	316	338	416	439
Oregon	213	266	288	248	221	216	221	270	284	282
Pennsylvania	1,875	1,957	1,813	1,677	1,370	1,257	1,289	1,358	1,556	1,697
Rhode Island	262	279	214	193	154	121	120	123	184	231
South Carolina	264	363	354	309	279	268	277	247	328	375
South Dakota	174	175	157	152	112	121	185	224	117	199
Tennessee	489	537	449	415	336	433	405	552	690	844
Texas	1,440	1,293	1,232	1,105	1,050	1,076	1,268	1,504	1,697	1,966
Utah	147	168	192	162	146	146	170	175	188	236
Vermon	75	72	78	71	46	32	48	37	56	50
Virginia	594	573	528	476	426	406	464	541	533	635
Washington	496	461	453	366	333	299	305	332	363	467
West Virginia	171	163	145	143	117	134	206	226	216	305
Wisconsin	898	948	945	728	548	592	626	682	713	883
Wyoming	36	52	39	23	34	47	33	51	55	55
American Samoa	0	0	0	—	—	—	—	—	—	—
Guam	0	0	0	—	0	20	0	0	7	16
Puerto Rico	685	625	553	572	626	569	527	465	412	438
Virgin Islands	0	4	7	9	3	4	6	6	4	5

[1] National and regional totals exclude American Samoa, Guam, Puerto Rico, and the Virgin Islands.
[2] Includes basic students only.

Table 30
GRADUATIONS FROM ASSOCIATE DEGREE NURSING PROGRAMS, BY NLN REGION AND STATE: 1984-85 TO 1993-94[1]

NLN REGION AND STATE	NUMBER OF GRADUATIONS									
	1984-85	1985-86	1986-87	1987-88	1988-89	1989-90	1990-91	1991-92	1992-93	1993-94
United States	**45,208**	**41,333**	**38,528**	**37,397**	**37,837**	**42,318**	**46,794**	**52,896**	**56,770**	**58,839**
North Atlantic	9,231	8,791	8,530	8,164	8,101	8,778	9,463	11,381	12,040	12,425
Midwest	12,679	11,512	10,418	9,734	10,050	11,234	12,343	13,656	14,767	14,884
South	15,454	13,744	12,794	12,570	12,884	14,851	17,264	19,524	21,656	22,926
West	7,844	7,286	6,786	6,929	6,802	7,455	7,724	8,335	8,307	8,604
Alabama	1,029	972	865	842	825	918	1,072	1,307	1,384	1,697
Alaska	40	23	25	20	30	30	30	45	30	33
Arizona	568	546	516	520	554	567	595	606	677	795
Arkansas	509	475	435	395	400	494	643	731	687	668
California	4,181	4,002	3,544	3,519	3,416	3,589	3,652	3,869	3,793	3,915
Colorado	351	294	342	342	345	349	454	481	498	505
Connecticut	377	310	309	282	227	281	300	405	380	376
Delaware	146	133	129	133	153	172	195	186	184	213
District of Columbia	59	38	61	55	55	45	44	18	26	34
Florida	2,505	2,315	2,017	2,143	1,944	2,098	2,457	2,790	3,037	3,243
Georgia	1,159	981	820	745	826	988	1,101	1,365	1,582	1,690
Hawaii	129	107	44	112	130	178	162	174	180	161
Idaho	224	218	178	202	182	214	220	256	244	252
Illinois	2,260	2,096	1,818	1,712	1,724	1,875	2,105	2,281	2,904	2,582
Indiana	1,098	1,078	984	845	952	1,034	1,199	1,289	1,405	1,507
Iowa	921	778	795	699	807	893	923	1,043	1,038	1,078
Kansas	603	511	470	519	521	809	808	772	776	769
Kentucky	1,096	789	773	783	851	922	1,116	1,315	1,530	1,637
Louisiana	344	344	326	328	295	341	452	574	847	902
Maine	189	161	163	122	151	162	186	235	285	342
Maryland	897	825	732	609	564	653	739	847	942	997
Massachusetts	1,055	995	1,129	942	890	904	1,048	1,100	1,222	1,346
Michigan	2,346	1,980	2,016	1,755	1,727	1,744	1,802	2,045	2,088	2,164
Minnesota	965	901	780	710	819	831	996	1,075	1,059	1,086
Mississippi	670	657	676	542	591	661	825	831	944	1,064
Missouri	866	804	677	666	686	775	943	1,100	1,111	1,347
Montana	78	83	71	59	69	88	107	103	106	115
Nebraska	247	65	56	41	72	80	131	193	255	235
Nevada	148	128	120	147	115	108	112	147	129	168
New Hampshire	203	187	179	179	189	237	250	282	384	365
New Jersey	1,026	975	820	794	783	904	947	1,139	1,211	1,220
New Mexico	296	321	357	314	368	492	453	475	497	508
New York	4,278	4,201	3,985	4,002	4,025	4,093	4,478	5,365	5,634	5,576
North Carolina	1,719	1,159	1,070	1,126	1,254	1,517	1,695	1,731	1,982	2,110
North Dakota	114	87	61	—	—	—	—	—	—	—
Ohio	2,114	2,199	1,926	1,868	1,896	2,163	2,281	2,585	2,720	2,706
Oklahoma	534	443	491	532	575	611	772	843	866	974
Oregon	544	474	460	507	422	481	449	506	554	500
Pennsylvania	1,567	1,466	1,450	1,412	1,347	1,655	1,607	2,231	2,338	2,417
Rhode Island	188	188	202	169	214	217	303	285	206	364
South Carolina	608	514	524	537	584	618	779	849	889	882
South Dakota	201	202	139	209	193	224	239	217	297	264
Tennessee	906	854	840	807	824	884	1,014	1,151	1,308	1,256
Texas	2,088	2,023	2,013	1,973	2,161	2,728	3,179	3,605	3,821	3,889
Utah	395	205	210	292	331	329	430	489	456	494
Vermont	143	137	103	74	67	108	105	135	170	172
Virginia	796	825	709	799	775	909	935	1,105	1,248	1,351
Washington	795	802	840	783	723	886	890	977	924	962
West Virginia	594	568	503	409	415	509	485	480	589	566
Wisconsin	944	811	696	710	653	806	916	1,056	1,114	1,146
Wyoming	95	83	79	112	117	144	170	207	219	196
American Samoa	11	10	10	10	10	12	13	12	6	6
Guam	12	12	12	—	—	—	—	—	—	—
Puerto Rico	601	392	492	336	336	453	462	449	539	477
Virgin Islands	12	9	5	8	8	2	6	8	6	9

[1] National and regional totals exclude American Samoa, Guam, Puerto Rico, and the Virgin Islands.

Table 31
GRADUATIONS FROM DIPLOMA NURSING PROGRAMS, BY NLN REGION AND STATE: 1984-85 TO 1993-94[1]

NLN REGION AND STATE	NUMBER OF GRADUATIONS									
	1984-85	1985-86	1986-87	1987-88	1988-89	1989-90	1990-91	1991-92	1992-93	1993-94
United States	**11,892**	**10,524**	**8,272**	**5,938**	**4,826**	**5,199**	**6,172**	**6,528**	**6,937**	**7,119**
North Atlantic	4,338	4,087	3,424	2,733	2,151	2,361	2,814	3,087	3,117	3,196
Midwest	5,050	4,266	3,028	1,908	1,458	1,450	1,757	1,721	2,006	1,973
South	2,192	1,944	1,633	1,130	1,080	1,263	1,429	1,528	1,597	1,774
West	312	277	187	167	137	125	172	192	217	176
Alabama	110	104	34	20	18	16	12	38	33	33
Alaska	0	0	0	—	—	—	—	—	—	—
Arizona	0	0	0	—	—	—	—	—	—	—
Arkansas	84	89	103	90	135	188	211	252	273	289
California	246	202	187	167	137	125	172	192	217	176
Colorado	66	25	0	—	—	—	—	—	—	—
Connecticut	267	244	203	165	176	196	223	186	153	155
Delaware	8	12	12	8	9	8	10	8	8	24
District of Columbia	0	0	0	—	—	—	—	—	—	—
Florida	137	110	77	51	57	66	107	87	73	87
Georgia	105	141	166	76	54	61	50	—	—	—
Hawaii	0	0	0	—	—	—	—	—	—	—
Idaho	0	0	0	—	—	—	—	—	—	—
Illinois	868	731	396	278	155	141	218	93	208	225
Indiana	294	253	258	136	81	72	50	23	35	55
Iowa	423	350	180	114	112	110	131	169	243	254
Kansas	135	93	37	33	10	17	20	24	—	—
Kentucky	0	0	0	—	—	—	—	—	—	—
Louisiana	194	218	222	181	194	167	156	26	35	37
Maine	39	47	25	—	—	—	—	—	—	—
Maryland	189	139	94	72	74	98	90	120	131	136
Massachusetts	649	508	395	291	164	224	286	325	366	379
Michigan	308	254	206	158	112	111	133	170	202	225
Minnesota	183	92	0	—	—	—	—	—	—	—
Mississippi	26	0	0	—	—	—	—	—	—	—
Missouri	623	623	465	379	339	358	495	404	489	422
Montana	0	0	0	—	—	—	—	—	—	—
Nebraska	308	278	222	62	57	40	40	53	57	61
Nevada	0	0	0	—	—	—	—	—	—	—
New Hampshire	38	23	14	29	—	—	—	—	—	—
New Jersey	597	678	630	502	440	418	525	623	708	761
New Mexico	0	0	0	—	—	—	—	—	—	—
New York	670	629	523	326	219	262	335	371	177	198
North Carolina	216	182	131	88	66	119	197	230	226	229
North Dakota	139	140	51	—	—	—	—	—	—	—
Ohio	1,425	1,268	1,103	687	557	555	614	753	730	691
Oklahoma	0	0	0	—	—	—	—	—	—	—
Oregon	0	0	0	—	—	—	—	—	—	—
Pennsylvania	1,999	1,881	1,581	1,370	1,118	1,227	1,419	1,552	1,674	1,649
Rhode Island	71	65	41	42	25	26	16	22	31	30
South Carolina	29	12	6	—	—	—	—	—	—	—
South Dakota	59	44	28	17	17	20	18	—	—	—
Tennessee	517	459	384	209	136	119	152	233	254	311
Texas	124	109	102	108	109	147	158	205	202	194
Utah	0	0	0	—	—	—	—	—	—	—
Vermont	0	0	0	—	—	—	—	—	—	—
Virginia	355	279	228	184	155	201	219	267	301	388
Washington	0	0	0	—	—	—	—	—	—	—
West Virginia	106	102	86	51	82	81	77	70	69	70
Wisconsin	285	140	82	44	18	26	38	32	42	40
Wyoming	0	0	0	—	—	—	—	—	—	—
American Samoa	0	0	0	—	—	—	0	—	—	—
Guam	0	0	0	—	—	—	0	—	—	—
Puerto Rico	0	0	0	—	—	—	0	—	—	—
Virgin Islands	0	0	0	—	—	—	0	—	—	—

[1] National and regional totals exclude American Samoa, Guam, Puerto Rico, and the Virgin Islands.

Table 32
BASIC AND RN STUDENT GRADUATIONS FROM BACCALAUREATE NURSING PROGRAMS: 1984-85 TO 1993-94[1]

| YEAR | GRADUATIONS FROM BACCALAUREATE NURSING PROGRAMS | | | |
| | Total Graduations | Basic Programs | | BRN* Programs |
		Basic Students	RN Students	RN Students
1984-85	34,569	24,975	5,587	4,007
1985-86	35,550	25,170	5,698	4,682
1986-87	34,475	23,761	6,591	4,123
1987-88	32,672	21,504	6,710	4,458
1988-89	30,543	18,997	7,195	4,351
1989-90	30,763	18,571	7,241	4,951
1990-91	29,438	19,264	7,027	3,147
1991-92	32,029	21,415	7,064	3,550
1992-93	34,504	24,442	6,360	3,702
1993-94	39,693	28,912	7,018	3,763

[1] Excludes American Samoa, Guam, Puerto Rico, and the Virgin Islands.
* BRN programs are baccalaureate programs that admit only RNs.

Table 33
GRADUATIONS OF REGISTERED NURSES FROM BACCALAUREATE NURSING PROGRAMS, BY PREVIOUS BASIC NURSING EDUCATION AND REGION: 1989-90 TO 1993-94[1]

| YEAR AND REGION | BACCALAUREATE PROGRAMS ACCEPTING RNs | PREVIOUS NURSING CREDENTIAL[2] | | |
		Total	Diploma	Associate Degree
1989-90 (Total)	**628**	**12,192**	**4,323**	**7,869**
North Atlantic	154	2,998	1,226	1,772
Midwest	197	4,152	1,799	2,353
South	199	3,046	840	2,206
West	78	1,996	458	1,538
1990-91 (Total)	**667**	**10,174**	**3,679**	**6,495**
North Atlantic	159	2,886	1,179	1,707
Midwest	213	3,054	1,415	1,639
South	215	2,855	770	2,085
West	80	1,379	315	1,064
1991-92 (Total)	**637**	**10,614**	**3,691**	**6,923**
North Atlantic	158	2,963	1,289	1,674
Midwest	197	3,282	1,298	1,984
South	205	2,926	808	2,118
West	77	1,443	296	1,147
1992-93 (Total)	**644**	**10,062**	**3,083**	**6,979**
North Atlantic	164	2,741	1,114	1,627
Midwest	201	2,924	1,062	1,862
South	206	2,711	627	2,084
West	73	1,686	280	1,406
1993-94 (Total)	**646**	**10,781**	**3,792**	**6,989**
North Atlantic	166	3,160	1,377	1,783
Midwest	200	3,133	1,400	1,733
South	207	3,075	760	2,315
West	73	1,413	255	1,158

[1] Excludes American Samoa, Guam, Puerto Rico, and the Virgin Islands.
[2] Includes RNs in basic programs, RNs in BRN programs, and basic BSN students.

Table 34

TOTAL GRADUATIONS FROM BACCALAUREATE NURSING PROGRAMS, BY NLN REGION AND STATE:
1990 TO 1994[1]

NLN REGION AND STATE	GRADUATIONS FROM BACCALAUREATE NURSING PROGRAMS [2]									
	1990		1991		1992		1993		1994	
	Total	RNs Only	Total	RNs Only	Total	RNs Only	Total	RNs Only	Total	RNs Only
United States	**30,763**	**12,192**	**29,438**	**10,174**	**32,029**	**10,614**	**34,504**	**10,062**	**39,693**	**10,781**
North Atlantic	7,206	2,998	6,887	2,886	7,257	2,963	7,700	2,741	8,953	3,160
Midwest	9,822	4,152	8,915	3,054	9,805	3,282	10,288	2,924	11,989	3,133
South	8,914	3,046	9,376	2,855	10,496	2,926	11,505	2,711	13,508	3,075
West	4,821	1,996	4,260	1,379	4,471	1,443	5,011	1,686	5,243	1,413
Alabama	763	272	720	239	773	251	751	198	1,141	229
Alaska	39	7	37	16	44	12	59	11	51	5
Arizona	747	507	556	355	388	202	546	305	587	318
Arkansas	233	37	225	40	274	33	297	41	357	60
California	2,109	867	1,629	408	1,789	605	1,988	703	1,796	296
Colorado	358	123	428	131	497	133	614	200	596	135
Connecticut	346	113	332	118	422	135	424	146	464	172
Delaware	146	53	122	55	144	54	181	96	214	93
District of Columbia	174	28	158	33	216	46	175	20	237	37
Florida	897	384	929	429	1,044	425	1,107	383	1,177	482
Georgia	614	217	627	174	649	166	756	174	1,003	226
Hawaii	168	96	215	81	174	108	168	72	157	59
Idaho	119	63	117	46	103	23	130	56	127	54
Illinois	1,523	594	1,397	556	1,322	430	1,478	459	1,745	400
Indiana	940	299	897	265	1,020	298	1,018	222	1,291	316
Iowa	818	587	396	157	461	190	443	139	481	157
Kansas	495	150	541	155	521	126	639	103	705	115
Kentucky	542	211	489	181	541	182	581	117	658	105
Louisiana	540	68	693	85	692	91	898	80	960	88
Maine	138	31	158	18	201	36	230	32	288	36
Maryland	495	233	512	234	671	315	664	274	795	263
Massachusetts	966	368	925	394	961	370	988	304	1,203	392
Michigan	1,496	768	1,192	439	1,357	556	1,537	568	1,412	479
Minnesota	522	183	529	140	599	172	710	170	831	253
Mississippi	344	94	392	70	455	60	502	77	574	67
Missouri	745	422	639	306	812	353	921	346	1,157	447
Montana	143	6	106	6	154	14	120	11	164	12
Nebraska	402	175	401	142	525	158	490	99	643	95
Nevada	79	34	93	32	104	15	116	17	117	19
New Hampshire	104	28	113	32	111	34	176	57	184	64
New Jersey	609	291	570	276	515	250	572	233	664	273
New Mexico	99	41	113	67	119	60	149	80	184	91
New York	2,341	1,114	2,160	1,068	2,164	1,033	2,372	1,067	2,687	1,059
North Carolina	581	212	655	205	865	279	988	286	1,088	364
North Dakota	228	42	262	47	305	34	334	46	354	60
Ohio	1,580	572	1,540	537	1,603	591	1,636	520	2,050	573
Oklahoma	356	86	436	120	427	89	499	83	498	59
Oregon	277	61	285	64	328	58	295	11	345	63
Pennsylvania	2,164	907	2,107	818	2,289	931	2,268	712	2,605	908
Rhode Island	167	46	160	40	170	47	234	50	324	93
South Carolina	394	126	411	134	324	77	452	124	476	101
South Dakota	164	43	231	46	293	69	174	57	252	53
Tennessee	697	264	605	200	801	249	934	244	1,067	223
Texas	1,510	434	1,681	413	1,889	385	2,051	354	2,401	435
Utah	234	88	223	53	247	72	262	74	345	109
Vermont	51	19	82	34	64	27	80	24	83	33
Virginia	655	249	708	244	789	248	758	225	914	279
Washington	386	87	418	113	454	122	505	142	716	249
West Virginia	293	159	293	87	302	76	267	51	399	94
Wisconsin	909	317	890	264	987	305	908	195	1,068	185
Wyoming	63	16	40	7	70	19	59	4	58	3
American Samoa	—	—	—	—	—	—	—	—	—	—
Guam	20	—	5	5	0	0	14	7	16	0
Puerto Rico	708	139	678	151	598	133	620	208	572	134
Virgin Islands	7	3	7	1	7	1	6	2	11	6

[1] National and regional totals exclude American Samoa, Guam, Puerto Rico, and the Virgin Islands.
[2] Totals include RNs in basic programs, RNs in BRN programs, and basic BSN students.

Table 35
APPLICATIONS PER FALL ADMISSION FOR BASIC RN PROGRAMS, BY TYPE OF PROGRAM AND NLN REGION: 1994

NLN REGION	NUMBER OF APPLICATIONS	NUMBER OF FALL ADMISSIONS	APPLICATIONS PER FALL ADMISSIONS
ALL REPORTING RN PROGRAMS[2]			
All Regions	257,797	85,653	3.01
North Atlantic	70,532	23,477	3.00
Midwest	62,833	22,780	2.76
South	95,324	30,830	3.09
West	29,108	8,566	3.40
BACCALAUREATE PROGRAMS			
All Regions	82,435	30,246	2.72
North Atlantic	23,604	7,469	3.16
Midwest	22,114	9,535	2.32
South	27,286	10,140	2.69
West	9,431	3,102	3.04
ASSOCIATE DEGREE PROGRAMS			
All Regions	155,161	48,598	3.19
North Atlantic	36,500	12,686	2.88
Midwest	35,588	11,650	3.05
South	63,684	18,875	3.37
West	19,389	5,387	3.60
DIPLOMA PROGRAMS			
All Regions	20,201	6,809	2.97
North Atlantic	10,428	3,322	3.14
Midwest	5,131	1,595	3.22
South	4,354	1,815	2.40
West	288	77	3.74

[1] Excludes American Samoa, Guam, Puerto Rico and the Virgin Islands.

[2] To be included in this tabulation, a nursing program must have answered the question on number of applications and must have admitted a class in the fall of the survey year.

Table 36
PERCENTAGE OF APPLICATIONS FOR ADMISSION ACCEPTED AND NOT ACCEPTED AND PERCENTAGE ON WAITING LISTS FOR ALL BASIC RN PROGRAMS, BY TYPE OF PROGRAM: 1994

ALL REPORTING RN PROGRAMS	
Total applications	100.0
Accepted	43.0
Not accepted	57.0
Percent of qualified applicants not accepted and placed on waiting lists.	20.3
BACCALAUREATE PROGRAMS	
Total applications	100.0
Accepted	50.5
Not accepted	49.5
Percent of qualified applicants not accepted and placed on waiting lists.	17.9
ASSOCIATE DEGREE PROGRAMS	
Total applications	100.0
Accepted	38.6
Not accepted	61.4
Percent of qualified applicants not accepted and placed on waiting lists.	22.9
DIPLOMA PROGRAMS	
Total applications	100.0
Accepted	45.4
Not accepted	54.6
Percent of qualified applicants not accepted and placed on waiting lists.	10.7

Section 4
Numeric Tables
on Male and Minority Students

Table 1
ESTIMATED NUMBER OF STUDENT ADMISSIONS
TO ALL BASIC RN PROGRAMS, BY RACE/ETHNICITY, NLN REGION AND STATE: 1993-1994[1]

NLN REGION AND STATE	NUMBER OF PROGRAMS	TOTAL NUMBER OF ADMISSIONS[2]	NUMBER OF ADMISSIONS					
			White	Black	Hispanic	Asian	American Indian	Other/ Unknown
United States	**1,501**	**129,897**	**106,707**	**11,514**	**4,186**	**4,462**	**959**	**2,037**
North Atlantic	329	33,140	26,669	3,445	888	1,150	120	859
Midwest	434	34,840	31,102	1,862	515	789	203	351
South	513	46,979	38,347	5,475	1,521	882	348	403
West	225	14,938	10,589	732	1,262	1,641	288	424
Alabama	36	3,847	3,215	536	9	40	37	10
Alaska	2	110	89	4	5	5	4	3
Arizona	16	1,281	1,111	17	86	41	18	11
Arkansas	22	1,751	1,555	153	9	11	14	9
California	94	6,710	3,853	563	751	1,207	112	222
Colorado	17	1,041	818	49	128	19	11	15
Connecticut	17	1,049	888	89	40	17	3	12
Delaware	7	532	373	129	5	13	1	10
District of Columbia	5	355	201	114	10	28	0	1
Florida	40	4,835	3,538	655	430	143	26	42
Georgia	32	3,366	2,790	433	44	35	8	56
Hawaii	7	395	192	11	18	171	1	2
Idaho	7	352	325	2	8	10	4	3
Illinois	71	5,774	4,543	639	165	367	10	49
Indiana	46	3,257	3,024	101	45	24	9	52
Iowa	40	2,358	2,291	26	12	7	6	9
Kansas	30	1,603	1,464	48	33	36	16	6
Kentucky	34	2,757	2,652	60	16	19	7	2
Louisiana	23	3,156	2,495	536	55	36	10	24
Maine	15	602	586	2	2	5	1	6
Maryland	24	2,269	1,814	290	35	67	9	57
Massachusetts	43	3,386	2,825	202	71	55	2	231
Michigan	50	4,236	3,608	414	56	92	36	27
Minnesota	21	1,997	1,892	42	15	25	20	2
Mississippi	23	2,211	1,945	242	11	2	4	7
Missouri	46	3,380	3,053	208	34	43	17	27
Montana	5	387	335	5	7	5	24	11
Nebraska	13	1,051	992	16	19	10	5	5
Nevada	6	319	272	8	14	21	2	2
New Hampshire	9	543	526	3	1	3	2	8
New Jersey	37	3,631	2,612	474	140	284	7	113
New Mexico	16	824	541	15	167	10	61	28
New York	100	13,942	10,335	2,000	509	618	81	397
North Carolina	62	4,141	3,560	423	27	41	20	66
North Dakota	7	406	384	0	1	6	15	0
Ohio	69	7,374	6,701	328	85	128	30	102
Oklahoma	28	1,710	1,397	70	41	32	154	16
Oregon	16	938	784	10	14	37	17	76
Pennsylvania	84	8,142	7,516	372	83	104	15	48
Rhode Island	7	673	530	59	26	17	8	33
South Carolina	20	1,778	1,465	265	6	16	4	24
South Dakota	10	554	533	0	2	4	13	2
Tennessee	36	3,654	3,164	391	16	38	18	27
Texas	77	7,344	5,477	748	782	275	26	37
Utah	7	685	647	1	14	13	10	0
Vermont	5	285	277	1	1	6	0	0
Virginia	37	3,027	2,176	654	40	120	8	26
Washington	24	1,626	1,371	43	42	100	20	50
West Virginia	19	1,133	1,104	19	0	7	3	0
Wisconsin	31	2,850	2,617	40	48	47	26	70
Wyoming	8	270	251	4	8	2	4	1

[1] Excludes American Samoa, Guam, Puerto Rico, and the Virgin Islands.
[2] Due to rounding, the racial/ethnic estimations sometimes add up to slightly less than the true total.

51

Table 2
ESTIMATED NUMBER OF STUDENT ADMISSIONS TO BASIC BACCALAUREATE NURSING PROGRAMS, BY RACE/ETHNICITY, NLN REGION AND STATE: 1993-1994[1]

NLN REGION AND STATE	NUMBER OF PROGRAMS	TOTAL NUMBER OF ADMISSIONS[2]	NUMBER OF ADMISSIONS					
			White	Black	Hispanic	Asian	American Indian	Other/ Unknown
United States	**509**	**42,953**	**34,823**	**4,005**	**1,312**	**1,738**	**241**	**827**
North Atlantic	113	9,746	7,720	991	274	393	19	344
Midwest	160	13,154	11,694	523	236	418	84	198
South	177	15,299	11,901	2,352	456	392	68	128
West	59	4,754	3,508	139	346	535	70	157
Alabama	12	1,091	936	125	3	25	0	1
Alaska	1	78	62	4	4	3	4	1
Arizona	4	347	293	3	24	23	4	1
Arkansas	9	591	515	65	2	6	2	1
California	23	1,768	1,016	70	214	346	34	88
Colorado	7	506	436	20	34	12	1	3
Connecticut	8	456	413	21	4	12	2	4
Delaware	2	256	146	93	3	10	0	4
District of Columbia	4	293	198	57	10	26	0	1
Florida	13	940	602	206	84	39	2	7
Georgia	12	1,016	834	106	20	16	1	40
Hawaii	3	196	122	11	6	54	1	2
Idaho	2	90	78	2	2	5	2	1
Illinois	27	2,278	1,869	136	69	171	3	30
Indiana	20	1,338	1,234	44	17	13	3	27
Iowa	12	489	471	2	5	4	1	4
Kansas	11	694	617	22	16	25	8	6
Kentucky	10	785	736	27	13	8	1	0
Louisiana	13	2,086	1,562	446	31	26	6	15
Maine	7	237	225	1	1	5	0	5
Maryland	7	762	585	130	14	34	0	0
Massachusetts	15	1,227	950	77	27	24	2	147
Michigan	14	1,344	1,101	117	28	63	21	15
Minnesota	9	688	651	8	6	13	8	2
Mississippi	7	684	602	77	3	2	0	0
Missouri	15	1,262	1,175	40	20	19	2	8
Montana	2	258	223	4	7	5	8	11
Nebraska	6	745	703	10	18	8	1	3
Nevada	2	114	87	6	5	14	0	2
New Hampshire	3	162	150	1	1	2	0	8
New Jersey	7	562	350	94	32	45	2	38
New Mexico	2	128	96	5	18	4	3	2
New York	32	2,948	2,073	441	151	201	8	71
North Carolina	12	1,122	876	211	10	20	3	2
North Dakota	7	406	384	0	1	6	15	0
Ohio	22	2,272	2,008	123	19	63	4	55
Oklahoma	11	582	457	39	14	21	45	6
Oregon	3	376	321	3	7	21	4	20
Pennsylvania	31	3,259	2,929	196	38	58	4	34
Rhode Island	3	266	209	10	7	7	1	32
South Carolina	7	525	397	114	1	10	0	3
South Dakota	4	214	205	0	1	2	4	2
Tennessee	17	1,213	1,047	125	4	19	1	17
Texas	26	2,487	1,769	323	249	123	4	17
Utah	3	258	239	1	5	8	5	0
Vermont	1	80	77	0	0	3	0	0
Virginia	12	995	570	352	8	42	3	19
Washington	6	571	479	9	17	38	3	25
West Virginia	9	420	413	6	0	1	0	0
Wisconsin	13	1,424	1,276	21	36	31	14	46
Wyoming	1	64	56	1	3	2	1	1

[1] Excludes American Samoa, Guam, Puerto Rico, and the Virgin Islands.
[2] Due to rounding, the racial/ethnic estimations sometimes add up to slightly less than the true total.

Table 3
ESTIMATED NUMBER OF STUDENT ADMISSIONS TO ASSOCIATE DEGREE NURSING PROGRAMS, BY RACE/ETHNICITY, NLN REGION AND STATE: 1993-1994[1]

NLN REGION AND STATE	NUMBER OF PROGRAMS	TOTAL NUMBER OF ADMISSIONS[2]	NUMBER OF ADMISSIONS					
			White	Black	Hispanic	Asian	American Indian	Other/ Unknown
United States	**868**	**77,343**	**63,505**	**6,867**	**2,645**	**2,461**	**691**	**1,151**
North Atlantic	153	18,893	15,017	2,169	533	587	95	490
Midwest	241	19,356	17,290	1,233	249	326	110	131
South	309	29,071	24,184	2,889	983	470	269	275
West	165	10,023	7,014	576	880	1,078	217	255
Alabama	23	2,710	2,234	410	6	15	37	9
Alaska	1	32	27	0	1	2	0	2
Arizona	12	934	818	14	62	18	14	10
Arkansas	11	795	716	55	5	4	7	8
California	70	4,781	2,770	476	501	833	77	122
Colorado	10	535	382	29	94	7	10	12
Connecticut	6	413	313	60	28	4	0	8
Delaware	4	248	204	34	1	2	1	6
District of Columbia	1	62	3	57	0	2	0	0
Florida	26	3,798	2,900	434	305	99	24	35
Georgia	20	2,350	1,956	327	24	19	7	16
Hawaii	4	199	70	0	12	117	0	0
Idaho	5	262	247	0	6	5	2	2
Illinois	39	3,244	2,471	493	82	172	7	18
Indiana	25	1,849	1,720	57	28	11	6	25
Iowa	23	1,582	1,552	12	2	1	5	5
Kansas	19	909	847	26	17	11	8	0
Kentucky	24	1,972	1,916	33	3	11	6	2
Louisiana	9	1,014	883	87	21	10	4	9
Maine	8	365	361	1	1	0	1	1
Maryland	14	1,324	1,081	126	20	33	9	57
Massachusetts	21	1,634	1,381	109	38	25	0	81
Michigan	33	2,647	2,291	277	27	27	13	8
Minnesota	12	1,309	1,241	34	9	12	12	0
Mississippi	16	1,527	1,343	165	8	0	4	7
Missouri	27	1,658	1,458	155	12	15	13	5
Montana	3	129	112	1	0	0	16	0
Nebraska	6	248	236	3	0	2	3	2
Nevada	4	205	185	2	9	7	2	0
New Hampshire	6	381	376	2	0	1	2	0
New Jersey	14	1,652	1,222	209	59	101	4	56
New Mexico	14	696	445	10	149	6	58	26
New York	63	10,761	8,059	1,543	355	407	73	325
North Carolina	46	2,666	2,355	195	11	20	17	64
North Dakota	—	—	—	—	—	—	—	—
Ohio	34	4,214	3,866	162	59	60	23	44
Oklahoma	17	1,128	940	31	27	11	109	10
Oregon	13	562	463	7	7	16	13	56
Pennsylvania	23	2,813	2,624	105	31	32	7	12
Rhode Island	3	359	274	48	19	10	7	1
South Carolina	13	1,253	1,068	151	5	6	4	21
South Dakota	6	340	328	0	1	2	9	0
Tennessee	15	1,649	1,400	194	12	19	14	10
Texas	49	4,625	3,514	418	506	151	19	20
Utah	4	427	408	0	9	5	5	0
Vermont	4	205	200	1	1	3	0	0
Virginia	17	1,625	1,263	252	30	66	5	7
Washington	18	1,055	892	34	25	62	17	25
West Virginia	9	635	615	11	0	6	3	0
Wisconsin	17	1,356	1,280	14	12	13	11	24
Wyoming	7	206	195	3	5	0	3	0

[1] Excludes American Samoa, Guam, Puerto Rico, and the Virgin Islands.
[2] Due to rounding, the racial/ethnic estimations sometimes add up to slightly less than the true total.

Table 4
ESTIMATED NUMBER OF STUDENT ADMISSIONS TO DIPLOMA
NURSING PROGRAMS, BY RACE/ETHNICITY, NLN REGION AND STATE: 1993-1994[1]

NLN REGION AND STATE	NUMBER OF PROGRAMS	TOTAL NUMBER OF ADMISSIONS[2]	NUMBER OF ADMISSIONS					
			White	Black	Hispanic	Asian	American Indian	Other/ Unknown
United States	**124**	**9,601**	**8,379**	**642**	**229**	**263**	**27**	**59**
North Atlantic	63	4,501	3,932	285	81	170	6	25
Midwest	33	2,330	2,118	106	30	45	9	22
South	27	2,609	2,262	234	82	20	11	0
West	1	161	67	17	36	28	1	12
Alabama	1	46	45	1	0	0	0	0
Alaska	—	—	—	—	—	—	—	—
Arizona	—	—	—	—	—	—	—	—
Arkansas	2	365	324	33	2	1	5	0
California	1	161	67	17	36	28	1	12
Colorado	—	—	—	—	—	—	—	—
Connecticut	3	180	162	8	8	1	1	0
Delaware	1	28	23	2	1	1	0	0
District of Columbia	—	—	—	—	—	—	—	—
Florida	1	97	36	15	41	5	0	0
Georgia	—	—	—	—	—	—	—	—
Hawaii	—	—	—	—	—	—	—	—
Idaho	—	—	—	—	—	—	—	—
Illinois	5	252	203	10	14	24	0	1
Indiana	1	70	70	0	0	0	0	0
Iowa	5	287	268	12	5	2	0	0
Kansas	—	—	—	—	—	—	—	—
Kentucky	—	—	—	—	—	—	—	—
Louisiana	1	56	50	3	3	0	0	0
Maine	—	—	—	—	—	—	—	—
Maryland	3	183	148	34	1	0	0	0
Massachusetts	7	525	494	16	6	6	0	3
Michigan	3	245	216	20	1	2	2	4
Minnesota	—	—	—	—	—	—	—	—
Mississippi	—	—	—	—	—	—	—	—
Missouri	4	460	420	13	2	9	2	14
Montana	—	—	—	—	—	—	—	—
Nebraska	1	58	53	3	1	0	1	0
Nevada	—	—	—	—	—	—	—	—
New Hampshire	—	—	—	—	—	—	—	—
New Jersey	16	1,417	1,040	171	49	138	1	19
New Mexico	—	—	—	—	—	—	—	—
New York	5	233	203	16	3	10	0	1
North Carolina	4	353	329	17	6	1	0	0
North Dakota	—	—	—	—	—	—	—	—
Ohio	13	888	827	43	7	5	3	3
Oklahoma	—	—	—	—	—	—	—	—
Oregon	—	—	—	—	—	—	—	—
Pennsylvania	30	2,070	1,963	71	14	14	4	2
Rhode Island	1	48	47	1	0	0	0	0
South Carolina	—	—	—	—	—	—	—	—
South Dakota	—	—	—	—	—	—	—	—
Tennessee	4	792	717	72	0	0	3	0
Texas	2	232	194	7	27	1	3	0
Utah	—	—	—	—	—	—	—	—
Vermont	—	—	—	—	—	—	—	—
Virginia	8	407	343	50	2	12	0	0
Washington	—	—	—	—	—	—	—	—
West Virginia	1	78	76	2	0	0	0	0
Wisconsin	1	70	61	5	0	3	1	0
Wyoming	—	—	—	—	—	—	—	—

[1] Excludes American Samoa, Guam, Puerto Rico, and the Virgin Islands.
[2] Due to rounding, the racial/ethnic estimations sometimes add up to slightly less than the true total.

Table 5
TRENDS IN THE ESTIMATED NUMBER OF ANNUAL ADMISSIONS
OF MINORITY STUDENTS TO BASIC RN PROGRAMS, 1988-89 TO 1993-94[1]

YEAR	BLACKS		HISPANIC		ASIAN		AMERICAN INDIAN	
	Number	Percent	Number	Percent	Number	Percent	Number	Percent
ALL REPORTING RN PROGRAMS								
1988-89	11,705	11.4	3,287	3.2	2,646	2.6	545	0.5
1989-90	12,146	11.1	3,532	3.2	3,223	3.0	704	0.6
1990-91	10,822	9.5	3,619	3.2	3,536	3.1	840	0.7
1991-92	10,476	8.5	4,258	3.5	3,972	3.2	874	0.7
1992-93	11,064	8.7	3,834	3.0	4,144	3.3	812	0.6
1993-94	11,514	8.9	4,186	3.2	4,462	3.4	959	0.7
BACCALAUREATE PROGRAMS								
1988-89	3,303	11.4	892	3.1	850	2.9	153	0.5
1989-90	3,442	11.5	881	3.0	1,117	3.7	200	0.7
1990-91	3,363	10.0	1,053	3.1	1,336	4.0	265	0.8
1991-92	3,273	8.6	1,490	3.9	1,531	4.0	283	0.7
1992-93	4,011	9.7	1,079	2.6	1,664	4.0	211	0.5
1993-94	4,005	9.3	1,312	3.0	1,738	4.0	241	0.6
ASSOCIATE DEGREE PROGRAMS								
1988-89	7,228	11.3	2,084	3.0	1,549	2.4	370	0.6
1989-90	7,756	11.3	2,426	3.5	1,807	2.6	484	0.7
1990-91	6,521	9.3	2,327	3.3	1,920	2.7	552	0.8
1991-92	6,413	8.7	2,459	3.3	2,142	2.9	568	0.8
1992-93	6,406	8.5	2,509	3.3	2,159	2.9	575	0.8
1993-94	6,867	8.9	2,645	3.4	2,461	3.2	691	0.9
DIPLOMA PROGRAMS								
1988-89	1,175	11.7	310	3.1	247	2.5	22	0.2
1989-90	945	9.4	222	2.2	298	3.0	20	0.2
1990-91	937	9.2	239	2.3	285	2.8	24	0.2
1991-92	790	7.4	309	2.9	299	2.8	23	0.2
1992-93	647	6.4	246	2.4	321	3.2	26	0.3
1993-94	642	6.7	229	2.4	263	2.7	27	0.3

[1] Excludes American Samoa, Guam, Puerto Rico, and the Virgin Islands.

Table 6
ESTIMATED NUMBER OF STUDENT ENROLLMENTS
IN ALL BASIC RN PROGRAMS, BY RACE/ETHNICITY, NLN REGION AND STATE: 1994[1]

NLN REGION AND STATE	NUMBER OF PROGRAMS	TOTAL NUMBER OF ENROLLMENTS[2]	NUMBER OF ENROLLMENTS					
			White	Black	Hispanic	Asian	American Indian	Other/ Unknown
United States	**1,501**	**268,350**	**220,955**	**24,055**	**8,696**	**9,566**	**1,869**	**3,195**
North Atlantic	329	74,088	59,397	8,181	2,175	2,682	276	1,379
Midwest	434	71,004	63,340	3,797	1,061	1,712	364	720
South	513	94,284	77,481	10,680	3,113	1,784	669	549
West	225	28,974	20,737	1,397	2,347	3,388	560	547
Alabama	36	8,380	6,652	1,474	34	104	94	24
Alaska	2	269	225	8	7	9	17	3
Arizona	16	2,309	1,996	39	158	61	37	17
Arkansas	22	3,347	3,034	239	13	25	25	12
California	94	13,525	7,705	1,094	1,522	2,593	212	399
Colorado	17	1,903	1,644	64	133	35	16	10
Connecticut	17	2,796	2,408	198	85	59	9	37
Delaware	7	1,332	976	311	5	30	3	7
District of Columbia	5	1,051	797	112	29	95	3	15
Florida	40	8,918	6,607	1,132	846	249	34	48
Georgia	32	6,078	5,095	791	67	93	10	20
Hawaii	7	911	503	35	39	322	3	7
Idaho	7	704	667	1	13	13	7	3
Illinois	71	12,104	9,474	1,224	407	861	18	117
Indiana	46	7,370	6,816	275	80	64	25	110
Iowa	40	4,349	4,210	44	37	37	8	13
Kansas	30	3,072	2,824	97	55	52	27	16
Kentucky	34	5,594	5,372	134	23	37	9	18
Louisiana	23	10,130	8,174	1,545	148	118	58	87
Maine	15	1,934	1,885	9	10	13	7	11
Maryland	24	4,099	3,235	653	50	139	15	8
Massachusetts	43	8,334	7,252	534	152	160	19	217
Michigan	50	8,977	7,666	856	103	192	86	73
Minnesota	21	3,357	3,179	57	18	58	26	20
Mississippi	23	3,761	3,316	404	20	11	5	3
Missouri	46	6,017	5,485	319	57	69	10	76
Montana	5	915	863	9	9	7	26	1
Nebraska	13	2,458	2,291	46	56	45	7	13
Nevada	6	513	409	18	19	45	8	14
New Hampshire	9	1,418	1,369	11	6	18	6	8
New Jersey	37	7,698	5,273	1,104	407	707	24	183
New Mexico	16	1,428	958	26	263	20	134	26
New York	100	28,916	20,541	4,976	1,237	1,246	163	753
North Carolina	62	7,251	6,157	788	47	85	47	125
North Dakota	7	777	725	4	5	9	33	1
Ohio	69	14,487	13,233	682	134	199	39	199
Oklahoma	28	3,251	2,695	129	63	61	272	31
Oregon	16	1,680	1,509	17	40	75	32	12
Pennsylvania	84	18,009	16,616	791	188	283	27	105
Rhode Island	7	1,951	1,646	132	55	60	15	43
South Carolina	20	3,764	3,181	510	22	32	1	17
South Dakota	10	1,112	1,053	2	3	9	43	2
Tennessee	36	6,724	5,960	659	26	50	6	23
Texas	77	14,089	10,676	1,123	1,653	486	76	74
Utah	7	1,192	1,148	1	19	15	9	0
Vermont	5	649	634	3	1	11	0	0
Virginia	37	6,260	4,773	1,054	88	274	14	57
Washington	24	3,146	2,655	81	112	191	56	53
West Virginia	19	2,638	2,554	45	13	20	3	2
Wisconsin	31	6,924	6,384	191	106	117	42	80
Wyoming	8	479	455	4	13	2	3	2

[1] Excludes American Samoa, Guam, Puerto Rico, and the Virgin Islands.
[2] Due to rounding, the racial/ethnic estimations sometimes add up to slightly less than the true total.

Table 7
ESTIMATED NUMBER OF STUDENT ENROLLMENTS IN BASIC BACCALAUREATE NURSING PROGRAMS, BY RACE/ETHNICITY, NLN REGION AND STATE: 1994[1]

NLN REGION AND STATE	NUMBER OF PROGRAMS	TOTAL NUMBER OF ENROLLMENTS[2]	NUMBER OF ENROLLMENTS					
			White	Black	Hispanic	Asian	American Indian	Other/ Unknown
United States	**509**	**112,659**	**91,441**	**10,327**	**3,664**	**4,855**	**698**	**1,672**
North Atlantic	113	28,628	22,697	3,069	950	1,233	68	612
Midwest	160	33,649	29,523	1,682	609	1,108	181	545
South	177	38,817	30,966	5,161	1,247	997	222	223
West	59	11,565	8,255	415	858	1,517	227	292
Alabama	12	4,070	3,213	720	17	84	20	17
Alaska	1	212	172	8	6	7	16	3
Arizona	4	843	703	15	60	31	23	11
Arkansas	9	1,229	1,109	101	3	11	2	3
California	23	4,855	2,609	259	550	1,123	90	224
Colorado	7	981	837	39	60	28	9	8
Connecticut	8	1,463	1,306	60	28	41	1	27
Delaware	2	819	526	259	1	28	0	5
District of Columbia	4	955	719	103	25	92	2	14
Florida	13	2,328	1,569	346	303	97	5	8
Georgia	12	2,249	1,885	267	27	63	4	1
Hawaii	3	548	354	35	18	130	3	7
Idaho	2	215	193	0	7	8	6	1
Illinois	27	5,977	4,654	466	224	523	11	99
Indiana	20	3,614	3,277	167	35	45	10	80
Iowa	12	1,338	1,290	13	15	18	4	0
Kansas	11	1,613	1,472	47	22	41	16	15
Kentucky	10	2,013	1,898	62	17	19	1	16
Louisiana	13	7,280	5,832	1,186	96	87	42	37
Maine	7	1,305	1,264	5	7	13	6	11
Maryland	7	1,543	1,098	330	29	84	3	0
Massachusetts	15	4,000	3,378	251	75	99	16	181
Michigan	14	3,699	3,088	335	52	142	48	34
Minnesota	9	1,159	1,089	15	9	28	13	5
Mississippi	7	1,170	1,037	124	6	3	0	0
Missouri	15	2,527	2,271	117	40	35	3	61
Montana	2	622	588	3	6	4	20	0
Nebraska	6	1,872	1,726	40	50	42	4	10
Nevada	2	271	199	12	12	38	4	6
New Hampshire	3	582	558	2	3	11	0	8
New Jersey	7	1,672	1,004	281	129	190	4	64
New Mexico	2	352	241	9	74	11	17	0
New York	32	8,158	5,240	1,627	557	522	27	185
North Carolina	12	2,239	1,735	437	10	42	13	2
North Dakota	7	777	725	4	5	9	33	1
Ohio	22	6,313	5,609	334	65	122	10	171
Oklahoma	11	1,233	993	67	30	40	93	10
Oregon	3	773	698	6	18	40	9	2
Pennsylvania	31	8,405	7,567	447	106	198	9	78
Rhode Island	3	1,019	893	33	19	32	3	39
South Carolina	7	1,774	1,463	268	8	26	0	9
South Dakota	4	554	535	2	2	5	8	2
Tennessee	17	2,761	2,486	216	14	32	4	9
Texas	26	5,371	3,866	518	646	256	29	56
Utah	3	576	539	1	14	13	9	0
Vermont	1	250	242	1	0	7	0	0
Virginia	12	2,255	1,514	501	35	144	6	55
Washington	6	1,194	1,012	27	26	82	20	28
West Virginia	9	1,302	1,268	18	6	9	0	0
Wisconsin	13	4,206	3,787	142	90	98	21	67
Wyoming	1	123	110	1	7	2	1	2

[1] Excludes American Samoa, Guam, Puerto Rico, and the Virgin Islands.
[2] Due to rounding, the racial/ethnic estimations sometimes add up to slightly less than the true total.

Table 8
ESTIMATED NUMBER OF STUDENT ENROLLMENTS IN ASSOCIATE DEGREE NURSING PROGRAMS, BY RACE/ETHNICITY, NLN REGION AND STATE: 1994[1]

NLN REGION AND STATE	NUMBER OF PROGRAMS	TOTAL NUMBER OF ENROLLMENTS[2]	NUMBER OF ENROLLMENTS					
			White	Black	Hispanic	Asian	American Indian	Other/ Unknown
United States	**868**	**135,895**	**112,382**	**12,397**	**4,478**	**4,093**	**1,123**	**1,409**
North Atlantic	153	35,660	28,320	4,399	988	1,061	199	694
Midwest	241	32,385	29,263	1,921	368	494	167	163
South	309	50,773	42,445	5,131	1,715	727	429	318
West	165	17,077	12,354	946	1,407	1,811	328	234
Alabama	23	4,281	3,410	754	17	20	74	7
Alaska	1	57	53	0	1	2	1	0
Arizona	12	1,466	1,293	24	98	30	14	6
Arkansas	11	1,381	1,263	80	9	7	14	9
California	70	8,338	4,968	799	890	1,410	117	154
Colorado	10	922	807	25	73	7	7	2
Connecticut	6	976	788	111	46	13	8	10
Delaware	4	440	380	51	2	2	3	2
District of Columbia	1	96	78	9	4	3	1	1
Florida	26	6,399	4,967	756	463	144	28	39
Georgia	20	3,829	3,210	524	40	30	6	19
Hawaii	4	363	149	0	21	192	0	0
Idaho	5	489	474	1	6	5	1	2
Illinois	39	5,479	4,321	724	142	267	7	15
Indiana	25	3,493	3,296	92	42	18	15	30
Iowa	23	2,294	2,231	20	12	12	4	13
Kansas	19	1,459	1,352	50	33	11	11	1
Kentucky	24	3,581	3,474	72	6	18	8	2
Louisiana	9	2,769	2,267	356	49	31	16	50
Maine	8	629	621	4	3	0	1	0
Maryland	14	2,246	1,876	276	19	55	12	8
Massachusetts	21	3,148	2,776	230	62	46	2	32
Michigan	33	4,866	4,207	496	44	48	34	36
Minnesota	12	2,198	2,090	42	9	30	13	15
Mississippi	16	2,591	2,279	280	14	8	5	3
Missouri	27	2,689	2,447	182	14	25	5	15
Montana	3	293	275	6	3	3	6	1
Nebraska	6	483	468	3	4	3	2	3
Nevada	4	242	210	6	7	7	4	8
New Hampshire	6	836	811	9	3	7	6	0
New Jersey	14	2,909	2,128	382	117	206	17	59
New Mexico	14	1,076	717	17	189	9	117	26
New York	63	20,263	14,872	3,322	673	698	136	562
North Carolina	46	4,337	3,794	316	29	39	34	123
North Dakota	—	—	—	—	—	—	—	—
Ohio	34	6,283	5,862	269	51	59	21	22
Oklahoma	17	2,018	1,702	62	33	21	179	21
Oregon	13	907	811	11	22	35	23	10
Pennsylvania	23	5,146	4,831	182	41	56	13	24
Rhode Island	3	818	643	97	36	26	12	4
South Carolina	13	1,990	1,718	242	14	6	1	8
South Dakota	6	558	518	0	1	4	35	0
Tennessee	15	2,920	2,531	351	12	15	1	10
Texas	49	8,297	6,453	588	965	229	43	18
Utah	4	616	609	0	5	2	0	0
Vermont	4	399	392	2	1	4	0	0
Virginia	17	2,935	2,327	459	44	98	6	1
Washington	18	1,952	1,643	54	86	109	36	25
West Virginia	9	1,199	1,174	15	1	6	2	0
Wisconsin	17	2,583	2,471	43	16	17	20	13
Wyoming	7	356	345	3	6	0	2	0

[1] Excludes American Samoa, Guam, Puerto Rico, and the Virgin Islands.
[2] Due to rounding, the racial/ethnic estimations sometimes add up to slightly less than the true total.

Table 9
ESTIMATED NUMBER OF STUDENT ENROLLMENTS IN DIPLOMA
NURSING PROGRAMS, BY RACE/ETHNICITY, NLN REGION AND STATE: 1994[1]

NLN REGION AND STATE	NUMBER OF PROGRAMS	TOTAL NUMBER OF ENROLLMENTS[2]	NUMBER OF ENROLLMENTS					
			White	Black	Hispanic	Asian	American Indian	Other/ Unknown
United States	**124**	**19,796**	**17,132**	**1,331**	**554**	**618**	**48**	**114**
North Atlantic	63	9,800	8,380	713	237	388	9	73
Midwest	33	4,970	4,554	194	84	110	16	12
South	27	4,694	4,070	388	151	60	18	8
West	1	332	128	36	82	60	5	21
Alabama	1	29	29	0	0	0	0	0
Alaska	—	—	—	—	—	—	—	—
Arizona	—	—	—	—	—	—	—	—
Arkansas	2	737	662	58	1	7	9	0
California	1	332	128	36	82	60	5	21
Colorado	—	—	—	—	—	—	—	—
Connecticut	3	357	314	27	11	5	0	0
Delaware	1	73	70	1	2	0	0	0
District of Columbia	—	—	—	—	—	—	—	—
Florida	1	191	71	30	80	8	1	1
Georgia	—	—	—	—	—	—	—	—
Hawaii	—	—	—	—	—	—	—	—
Idaho	—	—	—	—	—	—	—	—
Illinois	5	648	499	34	41	71	0	3
Indiana	1	263	243	16	3	1	0	0
Iowa	5	717	689	11	10	7	0	0
Kansas	—	—	—	—	—	—	—	—
Kentucky	—	—	—	—	—	—	—	—
Louisiana	1	81	75	3	3	0	0	0
Maine	—	—	—	—	—	—	—	—
Maryland	3	310	261	47	2	0	0	0
Massachusetts	7	1,186	1,098	53	15	15	1	4
Michigan	3	412	371	25	7	2	4	3
Minnesota	—	—	—	—	—	—	—	—
Mississippi	—	—	—	—	—	—	—	—
Missouri	4	801	767	20	3	9	2	0
Montana	—	—	—	—	—	—	—	—
Nebraska	1	103	97	3	2	0	1	0
Nevada	—	—	—	—	—	—	—	—
New Hampshire	—	—	—	—	—	—	—	—
New Jersey	16	3,117	2,141	441	161	311	3	60
New Mexico	—	—	—	—	—	—	—	—
New York	5	495	429	27	7	26	0	6
North Carolina	4	675	628	35	8	4	0	0
North Dakota	—	—	—	—	—	—	—	—
Ohio	13	1,891	1,762	79	18	18	8	6
Oklahoma	—	—	—	—	—	—	—	—
Oregon	—	—	—	—	—	—	—	—
Pennsylvania	30	4,458	4,218	162	41	29	5	3
Rhode Island	1	114	110	2	0	2	0	0
South Carolina	—	—	—	—	—	—	—	—
South Dakota	—	—	—	—	—	—	—	—
Tennessee	4	1,043	943	92	0	3	1	4
Texas	2	421	357	17	42	1	4	0
Utah	—	—	—	—	—	—	—	—
Vermont	—	—	—	—	—	—	—	—
Virginia	8	1,070	932	94	9	32	2	1
Washington	—	—	—	—	—	—	—	—
West Virginia	1	137	112	12	6	5	1	2
Wisconsin	1	135	126	6	0	2	1	0
Wyoming	—	—	—	—	—	—	—	—

[1] Excludes American Samoa, Guam, Puerto Rico, and the Virgin Islands.
[2] Due to rounding, the racial/ethnic estimations sometimes add up to slightly less than the true total.

Table 10
TRENDS IN THE ESTIMATED NUMBER OF ENROLLMENTS
OF MINORITY STUDENTS IN BASIC RN PROGRAMS, 1989 TO 1994[1]

YEAR	BLACKS		HISPANIC		ASIAN		AMERICAN INDIAN	
	Number	Percent	Number	Percent	Number	Percent	Number	Percent
ALL REPORTING RN PROGRAMS								
1989	20,789	10.3	6,046	3.0	5,201	2.6	1,064	0.5
1990	23,094	10.4	6,580	3.0	6,591	3.0	1,803	0.8
1991	21,529	9.1	7,349	3.1	6,947	2.9	1,700	0.7
1992	22,147	8.6	7,667	3.0	8,306	3.2	1,685	0.6
1993	23,501	8.7	8,114	3.0	8,811	3.3	1,797	0.7
1994	24,055	9.0	8,696	3.2	9,566	3.6	1,869	0.7
BACCALAUREATE PROGRAMS								
1989	8,937	11.9	2,220	3.0	2,338	3.1	460	0.6
1990	9,610	11.7	2,519	3.1	3,160	3.9	586	0.7
1991	9,239	10.2	3,066	3.4	3,063	3.4	530	0.6
1992	9,154	9.0	2,896	2.8	3,966	3.9	663	0.6
1993	10,257	9.3	3,219	2.9	4,383	4.0	614	0.5
1994	10,327	9.2	3,664	3.2	4,855	4.3	698	0.6
ASSOCIATE DEGREE PROGRAMS								
1989	9,929	9.3	3,322	3.1	2,411	2.3	569	0.5
1990	11,593	9.9	3,568	3.0	2,930	2.5	1,025	0.9
1991	10,577	8.5	3,861	3.1	3,391	2.7	1,115	0.9
1992	11,327	8.5	4,237	3.2	3,687	2.8	976	0.7
1993	11,710	8.5	4,405	3.2	3,818	2.8	1,132	0.8
1994	12,397	9.1	4,478	3.3	4,093	3.0	1,123	0.8
DIPLOMA PROGRAMS								
1989	1,924	9.4	504	2.5	452	2.2	33	0.2
1990	1,891	8.6	491	2.2	504	2.3	190	0.9
1991	1,710	7.5	416	1.8	493	2.2	52	0.2
1992	1,666	7.2	534	2.3	653	2.8	46	0.2
1993	1,534	6.9	490	2.2	610	2.7	51	0.2
1994	1,331	6.7	554	2.8	618	3.1	48	0.2

[1] Excludes American Samoa, Guam, Puerto Rico, and the Virgin Islands.

Table 11
ESTIMATED NUMBER OF STUDENT GRADUATIONS FROM ALL BASIC RN PROGRAMS, BY RACE/ETHNICITY, NLN REGION AND STATE: 1993-1994[1]

NLN REGION AND STATE	NUMBER OF PROGRAMS	TOTAL NUMBER OF GRADUATIONS[2]	NUMBER OF GRADUATIONS					
			White	Black	Hispanic	Asian	American Indian	Other/ Unknown
United States	**1,501**	**94,870**	**81,449**	**6,455**	**2,841**	**2,796**	**566**	**726**
North Atlantic	329	21,414	18,243	1,816	454	593	65	238
Midwest	434	25,713	23,561	1,181	308	435	91	122
South	513	35,133	30,091	2,938	1,148	536	236	168
West	225	12,610	9,554	520	931	1,232	174	198
Alabama	36	2,642	2,331	267	2	16	14	12
Alaska	2	79	72	1	2	1	3	0
Arizona	16	1,064	944	14	62	16	8	23
Arkansas	22	1,254	1,149	86	3	13	3	0
California	94	5,591	3,549	408	556	916	43	118
Colorado	17	966	786	35	101	11	18	16
Connecticut	17	823	741	47	18	13	1	3
Delaware	7	358	302	18	18	17	2	1
District of Columbia	5	234	151	63	1	9	0	10
Florida	40	4,025	3,221	432	256	86	20	10
Georgia	32	2,467	2,136	271	17	28	3	10
Hawaii	7	259	102	3	13	139	0	0
Idaho	7	325	317	2	1	3	1	1
Illinois	71	4,152	3,422	372	121	206	5	25
Indiana	46	2,537	2,385	96	24	19	1	9
Iowa	40	1,656	1,601	17	4	9	1	21
Kansas	30	1,359	1,282	24	25	22	4	0
Kentucky	34	2,190	2,139	38	4	6	2	0
Louisiana	23	1,811	1,598	160	24	14	7	7
Maine	15	594	579	0	3	3	2	6
Maryland	24	1,665	1,406	202	11	40	2	1
Massachusetts	43	2,536	2,289	115	42	25	5	60
Michigan	50	3,322	2,925	287	37	43	12	14
Minnesota	21	1,664	1,618	14	11	12	11	0
Mississippi	23	1,571	1,397	166	4	4	0	0
Missouri	46	2,479	2,319	101	18	25	10	4
Montana	5	267	244	1	1	1	18	2
Nebraska	13	844	792	12	14	12	3	10
Nevada	6	266	241	2	8	9	3	3
New Hampshire	9	485	462	6	3	5	7	2
New Jersey	37	2,372	1,798	240	95	198	3	37
New Mexico	16	601	435	10	109	9	26	10
New York	100	7,402	5,768	1,058	211	241	29	93
North Carolina	62	3,063	2,721	214	19	27	21	57
North Dakota	7	294	283	0	0	5	6	0
Ohio	69	4,874	4,578	188	30	53	9	16
Oklahoma	28	1,413	1,228	46	11	15	104	9
Oregon	16	782	710	9	13	19	23	8
Pennsylvania	84	5,763	5,402	215	46	66	9	24
Rhode Island	7	625	533	54	16	14	7	1
South Carolina	20	1,257	1,067	158	8	14	2	7
South Dakota	10	463	443	1	3	3	13	0
Tennessee	36	2,411	2,155	212	8	25	2	9
Texas	77	6,049	4,666	392	739	166	50	34
Utah	7	730	695	3	12	11	6	3
Vermont	5	222	218	0	1	2	0	1
Virginia	37	2,374	1,959	284	40	74	4	12
Washington	24	1,429	1,220	31	48	95	21	14
West Virginia	19	941	918	10	2	8	2	0
Wisconsin	31	2,069	1,913	69	21	26	16	23
Wyoming	8	251	239	1	5	2	4	0

[1] Excludes American Samoa, Guam, Puerto Rico, and the Virgin Islands.
[2] Due to rounding, the racial/ethnic estimations sometimes add up to slightly less than the true total.

Table 12
ESTIMATED NUMBER OF STUDENT GRADUATIONS
FROM BASIC BACCALAUREATE NURSING PROGRAMS, BY RACE/ETHNICITY, NLN REGION
AND STATE: 1993-1994[1]

NLN REGION AND STATE	NUMBER OF PROGRAMS	TOTAL NUMBER OF GRADUATIONS[2]	NUMBER OF GRADUATIONS					
			White	Black	Hispanic	Asian	American Indian	Other/ Unknown
United States	**509**	**28,912**	**24,567**	**1,912**	**870**	**1,116**	**133**	**307**
North Atlantic	113	5,793	4,759	549	150	211	16	108
Midwest	160	8,856	8,084	321	125	231	31	62
South	177	10,433	8,807	926	364	238	47	45
West	59	3,830	2,917	116	231	436	39	92
Alabama	12	912	812	89	1	8	0	2
Alaska	1	46	42	0	2	0	2	0
Arizona	4	269	238	5	15	8	2	2
Arkansas	9	297	279	13	0	5	0	0
California	23	1,500	911	78	140	302	13	57
Colorado	7	461	390	12	33	5	5	16
Connecticut	8	292	268	8	6	7	0	3
Delaware	2	121	82	6	17	14	2	0
District of Columbia	4	200	150	31	1	8	0	10
Florida	13	695	535	89	51	16	3	1
Georgia	12	777	654	94	9	16	0	2
Hawaii	3	98	42	3	3	49	0	0
Idaho	2	73	68	1	1	1	1	1
Illinois	27	1,345	1,133	68	49	84	1	11
Indiana	20	975	908	44	9	9	1	3
Iowa	12	324	305	1	1	2	1	14
Kansas	11	590	549	8	11	20	2	0
Kentucky	10	553	528	19	3	2	1	0
Louisiana	13	872	757	88	13	4	4	5
Maine	7	252	248	0	2	1	1	0
Maryland	7	532	434	60	7	30	0	0
Massachusetts	15	811	705	37	12	10	0	48
Michigan	14	933	789	87	19	32	2	3
Minnesota	9	578	564	3	4	5	2	0
Mississippi	7	507	438	63	3	3	0	0
Missouri	15	710	661	23	6	14	3	3
Montana	2	152	143	1	1	1	4	2
Nebraska	6	548	511	10	11	10	1	4
Nevada	2	98	88	1	2	7	0	0
New Hampshire	3	120	116	1	0	1	0	2
New Jersey	7	391	276	48	17	42	0	8
New Mexico	2	93	73	1	14	2	3	0
New York	32	1,628	1,123	319	73	86	11	14
North Carolina	12	724	611	75	9	18	7	4
North Dakota	7	294	283	0	0	5	6	0
Ohio	22	1,477	1,361	66	6	31	2	11
Oklahoma	11	439	379	22	6	11	21	0
Oregon	3	282	262	2	2	12	3	1
Pennsylvania	31	1,697	1,522	91	20	41	1	23
Rhode Island	3	231	219	8	2	1	1	0
South Carolina	7	375	314	47	1	6	0	7
South Dakota	4	199	194	0	1	1	3	0
Tennessee	17	844	762	59	4	15	0	4
Texas	26	1,966	1,479	145	245	73	9	14
Utah	3	236	221	0	5	7	2	1
Vermont	1	50	50	0	0	0	0	0
Virginia	12	635	533	57	11	25	2	6
Washington	6	467	386	11	12	42	4	12
West Virginia	9	305	292	6	1	6	0	0
Wisconsin	13	883	826	11	8	18	7	13
Wyoming	1	55	53	1	1	0	0	0

[1] Excludes American Samoa, Guam, Puerto Rico, and the Virgin Islands.

[2] Due to rounding, the racial/ethnic estimations sometimes add up to slightly less than the true total.

Table 13
ESTIMATED NUMBER OF STUDENT GRADUATIONS FROM ASSOCIATE DEGREE NURSING PROGRAMS, BY RACE/ETHNICITY, NLN REGION AND STATE: 1993-1994[1]

NLN REGION AND STATE	NUMBER OF PROGRAMS	TOTAL NUMBER OF GRADUATIONS[2]	NUMBER OF GRADUATIONS					
			White	Black	Hispanic	Asian	American Indian	Other/ Unknown
United States	**868**	**58,839**	**50,602**	**4,150**	**1,790**	**1,475**	**409**	**385**
North Atlantic	153	12,425	10,621	1,092	251	295	43	120
Midwest	241	14,844	13,642	796	164	168	47	54
South	309	22,926	19,763	1,872	714	266	187	114
West	165	8,604	6,576	390	661	746	132	97
Alabama	23	1,697	1,486	178	1	8	14	10
Alaska	1	33	30	1	0	1	1	0
Arizona	12	795	706	9	47	8	6	21
Arkansas	11	668	616	42	0	7	3	0
California	70	3,915	2,577	316	377	564	27	52
Colorado	10	505	396	23	68	6	13	0
Connecticut	6	376	334	28	8	5	1	0
Delaware	4	213	199	10	0	3	0	1
District of Columbia	1	34	1	32	0	1	0	0
Florida	26	3,243	2,654	325	174	64	17	9
Georgia	20	1,690	1,482	177	8	12	3	8
Hawaii	4	161	60	0	10	90	0	0
Idaho	5	252	249	1	0	2	0	0
Illinois	39	2,582	2,101	297	62	105	4	11
Indiana	25	1,507	1,422	52	15	10	0	6
Iowa	23	1,078	1,052	10	2	4	0	7
Kansas	19	769	733	16	14	2	2	0
Kentucky	24	1,637	1,611	19	1	4	1	0
Louisiana	9	902	805	72	10	10	3	2
Maine	8	342	331	0	1	2	1	6
Maryland	14	997	859	121	3	9	2	1
Massachusetts	21	1,346	1,229	62	28	12	3	12
Michigan	33	2,164	1,939	183	15	7	7	10
Minnesota	12	1,086	1,054	11	7	7	9	0
Mississippi	16	1,064	959	103	1	1	0	0
Missouri	27	1,347	1,247	76	11	7	3	1
Montana	3	115	101	0	0	0	14	0
Nebraska	6	235	222	2	3	1	1	6
Nevada	4	168	153	1	6	2	3	3
New Hampshire	6	365	346	5	3	4	7	0
New Jersey	14	1,220	962	102	47	84	1	23
New Mexico	14	508	362	9	95	7	23	10
New York	63	5,576	4,468	731	134	149	18	76
North Carolina	46	2,110	1,895	127	9	8	14	53
North Dakota	—	—	—	—	—	—	—	—
Ohio	34	2,706	2,575	90	20	15	2	4
Oklahoma	17	974	849	24	5	4	83	9
Oregon	13	500	448	7	11	7	20	7
Pennsylvania	23	2,417	2,297	78	15	20	6	0
Rhode Island	3	364	286	44	14	13	6	1
South Carolina	13	882	753	111	7	8	2	0
South Dakota	6	264	249	1	2	2	10	0
Tennessee	15	1,256	1,104	135	4	10	1	2
Texas	49	3,889	3,032	237	468	91	40	20
Utah	4	494	474	3	7	4	4	2
Vermont	4	172	168	0	1	2	0	1
Virginia	17	1,351	1,101	198	22	28	2	0
Washington	18	962	834	20	36	53	17	2
West Virginia	9	566	557	3	1	2	2	0
Wisconsin	17	1,146	1,048	58	13	8	9	9
Wyoming	7	196	186	0	4	2	4	0

[1] Excludes American Samoa, Guam, Puerto Rico, and the Virgin Islands.
[2] Due to rounding, the racial/ethnic estimations sometimes add up to slightly less than the true total.

63

Table 14
ESTIMATED NUMBER OF STUDENT GRADUATIONS FROM DIPLOMA NURSING PROGRAMS, BY RACE/ETHNICITY, NLN REGION AND STATE: 1993-1994[1]

NLN REGION AND STATE	NUMBER OF PROGRAMS	TOTAL NUMBER OF GRADUATIONS[2]	NUMBER OF GRADUATIONS					
			White	Black	Hispanic	Asian	American Indian	Other/ Unknown
United States	**124**	**7,119**	**6,280**	**393**	**181**	**205**	**24**	**34**
North Atlantic	63	3,196	2,863	175	53	87	6	10
Midwest	33	1,973	1,835	64	19	36	13	6
South	27	1,774	1,521	140	70	32	2	9
West	1	176	61	14	39	50	3	9
Alabama	1	33	33	0	0	0	0	0
Alaska	—	—	—	—	—	—	—	—
Arizona	—	—	—	—	—	—	—	—
Arkansas	2	289	254	31	3	1	0	0
California	1	176	61	14	39	50	3	9
Colorado	—	—	—	—	—	—	—	—
Connecticut	3	155	139	11	4	1	0	0
Delaware	1	24	21	2	1	0	0	0
District of Columbia	—	—	—	—	—	—	—	—
Florida	1	87	32	18	31	6	0	0
Georgia	—	—	—	—	—	—	—	—
Hawaii	—	—	—	—	—	—	—	—
Idaho	—	—	—	—	—	—	—	—
Illinois	5	225	188	7	10	17	0	3
Indiana	1	55	55	0	0	0	0	0
Iowa	5	254	244	6	1	3	0	0
Kansas	—	—	—	—	—	—	—	—
Kentucky	—	—	—	—	—	—	—	—
Louisiana	1	37	36	0	1	0	0	0
Maine	—	—	—	—	—	—	—	—
Maryland	3	136	113	21	1	1	0	0
Massachusetts	7	379	355	16	2	3	2	0
Michigan	3	225	197	17	3	4	3	1
Minnesota	—	—	—	—	—	—	—	—
Mississippi	—	—	—	—	—	—	—	—
Missouri	4	422	411	2	1	4	4	0
Montana	—	—	—	—	—	—	—	—
Nebraska	1	61	59	0	0	1	1	0
Nevada	—	—	—	—	—	—	—	—
New Hampshire	—	—	—	—	—	—	—	—
New Jersey	16	761	560	90	31	72	2	6
New Mexico	—	—	—	—	—	—	—	—
New York	5	198	177	8	4	6	0	3
North Carolina	4	229	215	12	1	1	0	0
North Dakota	—	—	—	—	—	—	—	—
Ohio	13	691	642	32	4	7	5	1
Oklahoma	—	—	—	—	—	—	—	—
Oregon	—	—	—	—	—	—	—	—
Pennsylvania	30	1,649	1,583	46	11	5	2	1
Rhode Island	1	30	28	2	0	0	0	0
South Carolina	—	—	—	—	—	—	—	—
South Dakota	—	—	—	—	—	—	—	—
Tennessee	4	311	289	18	0	0	1	3
Texas	2	194	155	10	26	2	1	0
Utah	—	—	—	—	—	—	—	—
Vermont	—	—	—	—	—	—	—	—
Virginia	8	388	325	29	7	21	0	6
Washington	—	—	—	—	—	—	—	—
West Virginia	1	70	69	1	0	0	0	0
Wisconsin	1	40	39	0	0	0	0	1
Wyoming	—	—	—	—	—	—	—	—

[1] Excludes American Samoa, Guam, Puerto Rico, and the Virgin Islands.
[2] Due to rounding, the racial/ethnic estimations sometimes add up to slightly less than the true total.

Table 15
TRENDS IN THE ESTIMATED NUMBER OF GRADUATIONS
OF MINORITY STUDENTS FROM BASIC RN PROGRAMS, 1988-89 TO 1993-94[1]

YEAR	BLACKS		HISPANIC		ASIAN		AMERICAN INDIAN	
	Number	Percent	Number	Percent	Number	Percent	Number	Percent
ALL REPORTING RN PROGRAMS								
1988-89	5,698	9.2	1,882	3.1	1,180	1.9	317	0.5
1989-90	5,801	8.8	2,046	3.1	1,604	2.4	363	0.6
1990-91	5,350	7.4	2,026	2.8	1,809	2.5	363	0.5
1991-92	5,786	7.2	2,404	3.0	2,037	2.5	461	0.6
1992-93	6,024	6.8	2,340	2.6	2,270	2.6	610	0.7
1993-94	6,455	6.8	2,841	3.0	2,796	2.9	566	0.6
BACCALAUREATE PROGRAMS								
1988-89	1,765	9.3	575	3.0	435	2.3	113	0.6
1989-90	1,910	10.3	602	3.2	683	3.7	101	0.5
1990-91	1,552	8.0	525	2.7	765	4.0	115	0.6
1991-92	1,670	7.8	641	3.0	744	3.5	126	0.6
1992-93	1,799	7.4	587	2.4	918	3.8	193	0.8
1993-94	1,912	6.6	870	3.0	1,116	3.9	133	0.5
ASSOCIATE DEGREE PROGRAMS								
1988-89	3,588	9.5	1,170	3.1	675	1.8	197	0.5
1989-90	3,522	8.3	1,342	3.2	836	2.0	255	0.5
1990-91	3,415	7.3	1,307	2.8	937	2.0	236	0.5
1991-92	3,762	7.1	1,605	3.0	1,179	2.2	322	0.6
1992-93	3,860	6.8	1,584	2.8	1,211	2.1	405	0.7
1993-94	4,150	7.1	1,790	3.0	1,475	2.5	409	0.7
DIPLOMA PROGRAMS								
1988-89	347	7.2	137	2.8	69	1.4	7	0.1
1989-90	365	7.1	98	1.9	80	1.6	6	0.1
1990-91	381	6.2	196	3.2	109	1.8	11	0.2
1991-92	354	5.4	158	2.4	114	1.7	13	0.2
1992-93	365	5.3	169	2.4	141	2.0	12	0.2
1993-94	393	5.5	181	2.5	205	2.9	24	0.3

[1] Excludes American Samoa, Guam, Puerto Rico, and the Virgin Islands.

Table 16
ADMISSIONS OF MEN TO ALL BASIC RN PROGRAMS, BY NLN REGION: 1993-1994[1]

NLN REGION	NUMBER OF PROGRAMS REPORTING	TOTAL ADMISSIONS	MEN	
			Number	Percent
ALL REPORTING RN PROGRAMS				
All Regions	1,205	106,833	14,463	13.5
North Atlantic	275	28,364	4,011	14.1
Midwest	340	28,551	3,253	11.4
South	425	38,523	5,345	13.9
West	165	11,395	1,854	16.3
BACCALAUREATE PROGRAMS				
All Regions	399	35,189	4,369	12.4
North Atlantic	90	8,499	838	9.9
Midwest	122	10,725	1,241	11.6
South	143	12,314	1,744	14.2
West	44	3,651	546	15.0
ASSOCIATE DEGREE PROGRAMS				
All Regions	694	63,534	8,971	14.1
North Atlantic	131	16,239	2,619	16.1
Midwest	187	15,606	1,750	11.2
South	256	24,106	3,334	13.8
West	120	7,583	1,268	16.7
DIPLOMA PROGRAMS				
All Regions	112	8,110	1,123	13.8
North Atlantic	54	3,626	554	15.3
Midwest	31	2,220	262	11.8
South	26	2,103	267	12.7
West	1	161	40	24.8

[1] Excludes American Samoa, Guam, Puerto Rico, and the Virgin Islands.

Table 17
TRENDS IN ADMISSIONS OF MEN TO ALL BASIC RN PROGRAMS: 1984-1994[1]

YEAR	NUMBER OF PROGRAMS REPORTING	MEN	
		Number	Percent
ALL REPORTING RN PROGRAMS			
1984	1,348	7,971	7.0
1985	1,260	6,344	6.3
1986	1,228	5,715	6.6
1987	1,192	5,302	7.2
1988	1,257	5,958	7.3
1989	1,272	7,558	8.2
1991	1,194	10,033	10.7
1992	1,219	12,568	12.0
1993	1,243	14,111	12.9
1994	1,205	14,463	13.5
BACCALAUREATE PROGRAMS			
1984	404	2,384	6.4
1985	374	1,972	5.9
1986	382	1,783	6.0
1987	370	1,560	7.1
1988	412	1,675	6.7
1989	429	1,820	7.0
1991	412	3,003	10.4
1992	405	3,837	12.2
1993	412	4,434	12.6
1994	399	4,369	12.4
ASSOCIATE DEGREE PROGRAMS			
1984	695	4,712	8.0
1985	643	3,540	6.5
1986	643	3,432	7.1
1987	630	3,290	7.6
1988	682	3,726	7.6
1989	695	4,857	8.6
1991	654	6,089	10.9
1992	691	7,580	12.0
1993	711	8,357	13.1
1994	694	8,971	14.1
DIPLOMA PROGRAMS			
1984	249	875	5.1
1985	243	832	5.9
1986	203	498	5.3
1987	192	452	5.9
1988	163	557	6.8
1989	148	881	9.2
1991	128	941	10.1
1992	123	1,151	11.5
1993	120	1,320	13.6
1994	112	1,123	13.8

[1] Excludes American Samoa, Guam, Puerto Rico, and the Virgin Islands.

Table 18
ENROLLMENTS OF MEN IN ALL BASIC RN PROGRAMS, BY NLN REGION: 1994[1]

NLN REGION	NUMBER OF PROGRAMS REPORTING	TOTAL ENROLLMENTS	MEN	
			Number	Percent
ALL REPORTING RN PROGRAMS				
All Regions	**1,236**	**228,461**	**28,875**	**12.6**
North Atlantic	284	64,791	8,345	12.9
Midwest	358	61,152	6,233	10.2
South	427	79,864	11,125	13.9
West	167	22,654	3,172	14.0
BACCALAUREATE PROGRAMS				
All Regions	**418**	**97,744**	**11,717**	**12.0**
North Atlantic	93	24,883	2,484	10.0
Midwest	134	30,134	3,031	10.1
South	141	32,676	4,866	14.9
West	50	10,051	1,336	13.3
ASSOCIATE DEGREE PROGRAMS				
All Regions	**700**	**111,667**	**14,705**	**13.2**
North Atlantic	133	30,717	4,529	14.7
Midwest	191	26,048	2,637	10.1
South	260	42,631	5,801	13.6
West	116	12,271	1,738	14.2
DIPLOMA PROGRAMS				
All Regions	**118**	**19,050**	**2,453**	**12.9**
North Atlantic	58	9,191	1,332	14.5
Midwest	33	4,970	565	11.4
South	26	4,557	458	10.1
West	1	332	98	29.5

[1] Excludes American Samoa, Guam, Puerto Rico, and the Virgin Islands.

Table 19
TRENDS IN ENROLLMENTS OF MEN IN ALL BASIC RN PROGRAMS: 1984-1994[1]

YEAR	NUMBER OF PROGRAMS REPORTING	MEN	
		Number	Percent
ALL REPORTING RN PROGRAMS			
1984	1,348	13,652	6.2
1985	1,260	9,623	5.2
1986	1,228	8,259	4.4
1988	1,257	10,100	6.2
1989	1,272	12,404	6.9
1991	1,194	19,072	9.9
1992	1,157	22,823	11.1
1993	1,289	30,005	12.4
1994	1,236	28,875	12.6
BACCALAUREATE PROGRAMS			
1984	404	5,747	6.2
1985	374	3,787	4.9
1986	382	2,219	2.4
1988	412	3,363	5.4
1989	429	3,867	5.9
1991	412	6,973	9.8
1992	370	8,353	11.0
1993	438	12,470	12.3
1994	418	11,717	12.0
ASSOCIATE DEGREE PROGRAMS			
1984	695	6,052	6.5
1985	643	4,254	5.5
1986	643	4,992	6.7
1988	682	5,539	6.8
1989	695	7,033	7.5
1991	654	10,068	10.1
1992	669	12,178	11.2
1993	730	14,924	12.6
1994	700	14,705	13.2
DIPLOMA PROGRAMS			
1984	249	1,853	5.2
1985	243	1,582	5.5
1986	203	1,048	4.9
1988	163	1,198	6.5
1989	148	1,504	7.8
1991	128	2,031	9.6
1992	118	2,292	10.8
1993	121	2,611	12.2
1994	118	2,453	12.9

[1] Excludes American Samoa, Guam, Puerto Rico, and the Virgin Islands.

Table 20
GRADUATIONS OF MEN FROM ALL BASIC RN PROGRAMS, BY NLN REGION: 1993-1994[1]

NLN REGION	NUMBER OF PROGRAMS REPORTING	TOTAL GRADUATIONS	MEN	
			Number	Percent
ALL REPORTING RN PROGRAMS				
All Regions	**1,178**	**79,953**	**9,130**	**11.4**
North Atlantic	277	18,477	2,150	11.6
Midwest	323	21,266	1,998	9.4
South	414	30,099	3,630	12.1
West	164	10,111	1,352	13.4
BACCALAUREATE PROGRAMS				
All Regions	**393**	**25,350**	**2,816**	**11.1**
North Atlantic	88	4,977	442	8.9
Midwest	116	7,642	768	10.0
South	140	9,129	1,162	12.7
West	49	3,602	444	12.3
ASSOCIATE DEGREE PROGRAMS				
All Regions	**672**	**47,870**	**5,509**	**11.5**
North Atlantic	132	10,522	1,323	12.6
Midwest	175	11,699	1,018	8.7
South	251	19,316	2,295	11.9
West	114	6,333	873	13.8
DIPLOMA PROGRAMS				
All Regions	**113**	**6,733**	**805**	**12.0**
North Atlantic	57	2,978	385	12.9
Midwest	32	1,925	212	11.0
South	23	1,654	173	10.5
West	1	176	35	19.9

[1] Excludes American Samoa, Guam, Puerto Rico, and the Virgin Islands.

Table 21
TRENDS IN GRADUATIONS OF MEN FROM ALL BASIC RN PROGRAMS: 1984-1994[1]

YEAR	NUMBER OF PROGRAMS REPORTING	MEN	
		Number	Percent
ALL REPORTING RN PROGRAMS			
1984	1,348	4,286	5.8
1985	1,260	3,908	5.7
1986	1,228	3,916	5.5
1988	1,237	3,264	5.7
1989	1,272	3,080	5.7
1991	1,194	4,745	8.4
1992	1,006	6,178	9.9
1993	1,167	7,808	10.5
1994	1,178	9,130	11.4
BACCALAUREATE PROGRAMS			
1984	404	1,423	6.2
1985	374	1,198	5.6
1986	382	1,146	4.3
1988	393	983	5.2
1989	429	851	5.0
1991	412	1,201	8.2
1992	298	1,639	10.4
1993	376	2,233	10.5
1994	393	2,816	11.1
ASSOCIATE DEGREE PROGRAMS			
1984	695	2,325	5.7
1985	643	2,201	6.1
1986	643	2,326	6.8
1988	681	1,896	5.9
1989	695	1,989	6.0
1991	654	3,106	8.5
1992	609	4,027	9.7
1993	679	4,897	10.4
1994	672	5,509	11.5
DIPLOMA PROGRAMS			
1984	249	538	4.8
1985	243	509	4.5
1986	203	444	4.4
1988	163	385	6.7
1989	148	240	5.2
1991	128	438	8.0
1992	99	512	9.7
1993	112	678	10.6
1994	113	805	12.0

[1] Excludes American Samoa, Guam, Puerto Rico, and the Virgin Islands.

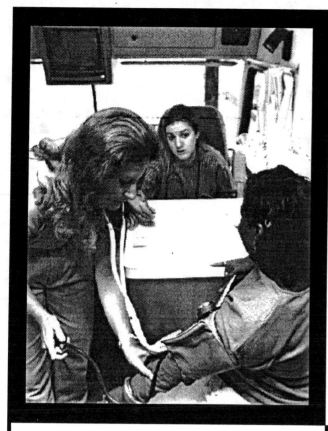
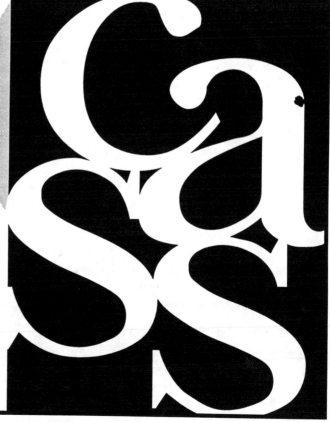

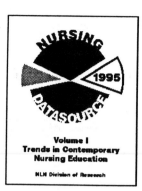

Nursing DataSource 1995

Nursing DataSource 1995 offers a comprehensive analysis of nursing education based on NLN's Annual Survey of Nursing Education Programs. The three volumes are devoted to contemporary nursing education, graduate education, and practical/vocational nursing, respectively.

Volume I—Trends in Contemporary Nursing Education
$35.00   *NLN Member Price $31.50*   Pub. No. 19-6649   ISBN 0-88737-664-9

Volume II—Graduate Education in Nursing: Advanced Practice Nursing
$35.00   *NLN Member Price $31.50*   Pub. No. 19-6657   ISBN 0-88737-665-7

Volume III—Focus on Practical/Vocational Nursing
$35.00   *NLN Member Price $31.50*   Pub. No. 19-6665   ISBN 0-88737-666-5

SPECIAL SUBSCRIPTION OFFER: Subscribe to *Nursing DataSource 1995*, **Volumes I, II,** and **III** for only $90.00—and save $15 over the single volume purchase price. *Sorry, no NLN discounts for this special offer (19-2705S).*

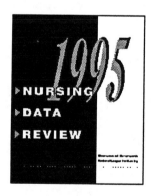

Nursing Data Review 1995

The most comprehensive research publication prepared by NLN Research, *Nursing Data Review 1995* compiles all the data from the Annual Survey of Nursing Education Programs and the Biennial Nurse Faculty Census. It is also the only source for complete statistics on faculty and students in practical and vocational nursing programs. Covering RN, LPN/LVN, and graduate nursing programs, this handy reference includes over 200 tables, figures, and maps, providing national, regional, and state indices on the nursing profession.

$37.95   *NLN Member Price $33.95*   1995   256 pp.   Pub. No. 19-2686   ISBN 0-88737-646-0

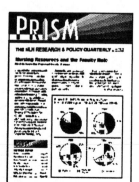

NLN Research & Policy PRISM

PRISM has quickly become one of NLN's most popular newsletters. Each volume is dedicated to a single emerging issue from the wide-ranging nursing and health care arena. *PRISM* is must-reading for anyone who needs an intelligent overview of nursing and health care trends.

One Year Subscription: $50   *NLN Member Price $45*   Pub. No. 19-2527S
Two Year Subscription: $89   *NLN Member Price $80*   Pub. No. 19-2554S

To order, use order form ▐▐▐▐▶

or call NLN Customer Service at 800/669-9656, ext. 138

ORDER FORM

Call Toll-Free (800) 669-9656, ext. 138, 9:00 a.m.–5:30 p.m. ET, Monday through Friday, or send this order form to: Customer Service, National League for Nursing, 350 Hudson St., NY, NY 10014. Send Internet e-mails (queries only) to: CUSTSERV@NLN.ORG. Or **FAX** your order—(212) 989-3710. *Please note: prices may be subject to change.*

Member Prices already reflect 10% discount. Discount of videos for purchase only.

No. of Copies

_____ **Pub. No.** _____ **Title** _____ $ _____

_____ **Pub. No.** _____ **Title** _____ $ _____

_____ **Pub. No.** _____ **Title** _____ $ _____

_____ **Pub. No.** _____ **Title** _____ $ _____

_____ **Pub. No.** _____ **Title** _____ $ _____

_____ **Pub. No.** _____ **Title** _____ $ _____

	Shipping and Handling via UPS Ground		
Order amount	Charges	Order amount	Charges
Up to $10.99	$2.65	75.00–99.99	8.15
11.00–24.99	3.95	100.00–124.99	9.45
25.00–49.99	5.50	125.00–149.99	11.05
50.00–74.99	6.85	250.00 and up	15.75

Subtotal $ _____

Additional Discount (if applicable) $ — _____

Shipping and Handling (see chart) $ _____

TOTAL INVOICE $ _____

METHOD OF SHIPPING:

☐ **UPS**   ☐ **RUSH/UPS**
(Please call NLN to verify additional charges.)

SHIP TO:

_____
(name)   (position)

_____
(nstitution)

_____
(ddress)

_____
(ity, state, ZIP code)

Telephone _____
              (area code)   (number)

FAX _____
       (area code)   (number)

BILL TO (if different from above):

_____
(nstitution)

_____
(ddress)

_____
(ity, state, ZIP code)

Date: _____

METHOD OF PAYMENT (U.S. dollars only):

☐ Check or Money Order enclosed

☐ P.O. # _____

☐ CHARGE THE ABOVE TOTAL TO

☐ MasterCard   ☐ Visa   ☐ American Express

Account No. _ _ _ _ _ _ _ _ _ _ _ _ _ _ _ _ _

Signature: _____

Expiration date: _____

NLN MEMBERSHIP NO.

CUSTOMER CODE NO.

FOR INTERNAL USE ONLY: Invoice # _____

C.S. Operator: _____   **Person Placing Order:** _____